1/2017

mdy

D1453151

Prognosis: Poor

One Doctor's Personal Account of the Beauty
and the Perils of Modern Medical Training

FRANCES
SOUTHWICK, D.O.

Prognosis: Poor. One Doctor's Personal Account of the
Beauty and the Perils of Modern Medical Training

Frances Southwick, D.O.

2015.
First Edition.
BookBaby.

Credit to contributors, editors: Judith Avers, "Mustang" Sally Cooper, Linda Farin, Greg Gallik, D.O.,
Theresa Labreglio, Melissa Malone, Tomoko Sairenji, M.D., Shauna Southwick, Samuel E. J. Sperstad, and
Donna Wilkinson.

Dedication / Acknowledgements

This book is dedicated to family medicine residents and their support networks of family, friends, mentors and colleagues.

Special thanks to my family for the building blocks. To my fellow residents for the laughter and connection. To my patients who make each day more meaningful. To my social media friends for all the good questions and inspiration. To Samuel Shem for the nerve.

To those who encouraged me to be myself and to follow my nose to medical school, especially: Louise Breyer, William Farrett, D.P.M., Mark "The Coot" Johnson, Kim Lasko, Susan & Lonnie Losh, Sheryl O'Dell, Beth Schutt, Marie Shipley and Jim Zakely.

To Elli & Theresa, Tomoko & Vince, BeckyJo, Nance, Greg & Joe, Pittsburgh's independent music scene (musicians and supporters) Sally & Greg, Cec, Emily & Sheila, Rie, Alissa, Yewah, Linda, Dan & Grete and The Early Mays & family for the steadfast, reverberating friendship that kept (and keeps) me afloat.

To Cynthia Magistro, Ph.D. for teaching me how to walk this fine line.

Most of all, to my patient and loving wife, Judith Avers... for everything (multilevel support, kindness, tolerance, sustenance, music, love and more).

Special thanks to ALL my medical school and residency instructors, especially those who took extra time with me: Krishan Aggarwal, M.D., Richard Ajayi, M.D., Helene Bender,

M.D., John Capito, M.D., Bruno Casile, D.O., Zach Comeaux, D.O., Barry Coutinho, M.D., Christopher D'Amanda, M.D., Bob Foster, D.O., Greg Gallik, D.O., John Garlitz, D.O., Donna Knupp, M.D., Debbie Kortyna, P.A., Christopher Kubicki, M.D., Dan Lapp, M.D., Earl Lee, D.O., Jasbir Makar, M.D., Andrea Nazar, D.O., Phil Phelps, L.C.S.W., R.K. Prasad, M.D., Keith Sargent, D.O., Lisa Schlar, M.D., Madeline Simasek, M.D., Ben Skinker, M.D., Karen Steele, D.O., Lori Stiefel, M.D., and Jackie Weaver-Agostoni, D.O.

Table of Contents

FOREWORD

"No matter how much you do to support them, you can't change the fact that being a resident sucks."

I asked a highly respected faculty physician what I could do to help our family medicine residents, and this was his response.

As the Director of Behavioral Science Curriculum for a family medicine (FM) residency program over the past dozen years or so, I have sought ways to reduce the obvious high level of stress for residents. They are routinely subjected to long work hours with abrupt shift changes. They change assignments monthly, often working in multiple medical institutions where they are guests of sorts, and are met with varying degrees of welcome. They answer to countless professionals who often offer conflicting orders. These are just a few of the purely structural demands FM residents confront over the three year training program.

Medicine is a demanding profession and not for the faint of heart. We, the public, have a very high expectation of our doctors. And doctors generally have even higher expectations of themselves. Physicians must develop the ability to perform at a very high level even when tired, uncertain and facing emotionally charged situations. They must be the symbol and voice of reason at the thin line where life and death meet. They must maintain compassion and empathy while appearing steadfast, despite the suffering and chaos that too often surrounds them.

These circumstances encourage us to push residents to the edge of their limits, perhaps even slightly beyond. Maybe it is essential for physicians to learn how deeply they must reach into themselves in order to develop and condition both the physical and emotional stamina necessary to master its demands. Demands such as:

- Managing a first-time mother's unexpected miscarriage.

- Fearing responsibility for a poor patient outcome.

- Telling a patient for the first time that their mass is cancer and it has already spread (and remembering the look on her face as she learns this).

- Analyzing and sometimes suppressing the uncertainty aroused by a patient who wants narcotics. (i.e. "Is the patient truly in intense pain or is he/she manipulating me because they have an addiction?")

- Being yelled at by a patient, a nurse, an attending physician, and a senior resident (all in the same day).

The counterquestion remains: Can training push them too far? What happens when even the most talented and emotionally strong human beings are immersed in overwhelming life circumstances? What happens when they have been conditioned to believe the sense they are "losing it" is a sign of weakness or simply a part of the experience that must be endured?

This is one of the places Dr. Southwick's book takes us. She guides us through experiences some have never imagined and others do not wish to recall. She takes us there in a personal way. This is not, however, the only place she shows us.

She also shares the humor and the joys that inevitably accompany an intense emotional journey.

My recollections of Dr. Southwick as a resident are of a quiet, unassuming young woman who was filled with compassion. She was insightful and reflective of her work and of her life. She was an active member of the Depression Quality Improvement Group that I chaired, and a regular attendee at the resident support activities she describes in the book. I knew of the extraordinary stressors she was managing as a resident, as a wife, as a daughter, and as a friend. I did not fully appreciate her journey until I read this book.

Whether you are medical student, a resident, an attending physician, or a family member of a physician, you will appreciate it too. You will see yourself in the characters and you will be moved.

I kept wondering as I read, what else could I have done? What else should I be doing to support residents through experiences like ones described by Dr. Southwick? I know there is more to be done and I will keep searching.

Phil Phelps, L.C.S.W., M.S.W., B.C.D.

Director of Behavioral Science Curriculum
and Clinical Associate Professor

University of Pittsburgh Medical Center Shadyside Family
Medicine Residency Program

INTRODUCTION

I am an osteopathic family medicine physician. This means I am a D.O., a doctor of osteopathic medicine, not an M.D. Osteopathy is a branch of medicine that focuses on treating the "whole" person, not just symptoms, with particular emphasis on preventive care. There are many similarities between M.D.s and D.O.s. After graduating from college, we all attend four years of med school. We all complete residency programs in hospitals, often together. The difference between us is that D.O.s receive special training in the musculoskeletal system. We use our hands to diagnose and treat many ailments: neck pain, back pain, even menstrual cramps and constipation. We also tend to be primary care doctors (family medicine, internal medicine, pediatrics, OB/GYN), but can specialize in anything (surgery, radiology, etc.). Your own physician might be a D.O.

I completed my medical residency (capstone training to become a full-fledged, independently-practicing physician) in 2013, and decided to write about it.

Why?

When doctors talk about first-hand accounts of residency, we all refer to our bible — The House of God. Published in 1978, the book was written by Samuel Shem, a resident who had just completed his intern year at a famous and well-respected hospital, under the guise of being "fiction," but everyone in medicine knew it was real. It depicted in gruesome detail the difficulties of residency in the 1970s, which included sex scandals among residents and nurses, no work-hour rules, corrupt hospital bureaucrats, poor patient care and residents becoming desperately depressed. The book brought much-needed attention to the fact that medical training at that time was in a very poor state of health.

Though a few things may have changed since then (for one thing, work hours are now capped on paper at 80 hours a week), residency training can still be overwhelming for many medical students and residents. According to a New York Times article called "Why Do Doctors Commit Suicide?" (Sept. 4, 2014) by Pranay Sinha, a first-year resident at Yale-New Haven Hospital, "young physicians at the beginning of their training are particularly vulnerable: In a recent study, 9.4 percent of fourth-year medical students and interns — as first-year residents are called — reported having suicidal thoughts in the previous two weeks." (Sinha, 2014)

Other than the book The House of God and a smattering of others, there seems to be a void of personal accounts about residency. There should be a plethora! There is no shortage of TV dramatizations, but fictionalizations cannot replace real experience.

There are a few reasons books on the subject are rarely written.

- Doctors are busy.

- It's hard to write a book.

But I think the biggest reason is this:

- People don't like to revisit bad memories.

When one experiences a trauma, it is tempting to simply "put the past behind" oneself and hope not to discuss it further. In fact, after it's over, many physicians block out much of their training experiences. And that is a shame, because so many young medical trainees are struggling, and feel alone. And so many people (including those who enter medical school) don't know what it *really* takes to become a doctor.

The process of becoming a physician can breed fear, shame, and disconnection. These lead to a sense of unworthiness and hopelessness. These feelings, when combined with sleep deprivation and unrealistic performance expectations, can be life threatening.

With this book, I take a step in unveiling the ugliness and shining a light on connection — not only for residents, but for those in close relationships with residents. This book was written with good intentions. I had the privilege of working in a top-notch institution with caring instructors and classmates and a very supportive group of family and friends. I am grateful to each of them for helping shape me into the person (and physician) I am.

I have changed many names of those involved, as well as some key identifying characteristics of the people and the groups to which they belong. I have also changed a few residents' graduation dates to protect their identities. Otherwise, although I accept that my memory is fallible, this book is as accurate a depiction of my experience as I can portray. I have also provided background information to explain how one arrives at residency.

The journey of becoming a doctor brought me intense love and appreciation for my wife, shared moments of joy and grief with my patients, sleeplessness, confusion, frustration, accomplishment, camaraderie with my fellow learners, and profound despair. I am not the same person I was when I started medical training. No one is ever the same after they experience something profound. But this is different. My personality has been sanded down. I interact differently with my friends and family. I look at things differently. I am no longer just Frances. I am Dr. Southwick.

TIMELINE

AGE	LIFE EVENT
0	Birth
0-4	Preparing for Elementary School
4-11	Elementary School / Preparing for Junior High School
11-13	Junior High School / Preparing for High School
13-17	High School / Preparing for College
17-21	College / Preparing for Medical School
21-25	Medical School / Preparing for Residency
25-29	Residency / Preparing for After Residency
30 +	After Residency

HOW IT BEGAN

"When did you know you would become a doctor?"

As far back as I can remember. One of my earliest memories is from age 4. I was at the home of Fiona Black, a boisterous woman who ran a daycare center for my neighborhood (picture a bustling house with kid noises and a trampoline in a tiny tumbleweed town, Eastern Colorado). After snack time, I walked around the yard and collected the remnants of our most prized summer treats: brightly colored Popsicles. I imagined myself grown up and dressed in a white coat, working in the office of our local physician, Dr. Depough. I would pretend to lift the lid off a gleaming canister and use one of my Popsicle sticks as a tongue depressor. Unfortunately, my sticky trophies were confiscated by Fiona, so I can't repurpose them in my office.

I also remember Freddie O'Donnell, my childhood snake-, turtle- and mischief-hunting partner, returning from his entry-to-school checkup. On his arm he had a cartoon Band-Aid and boasted, "I got my shot!" I overheard his mother telling my mom that Freddie had cried and thrown a tantrum during the visit. I was shocked — why would anyone cry at Dr. Depough's office? The office where he palpated your neck, determining a diagnosis just with his hands, and later you were rewarded with bubblegum-flavored amoxicillin you sipped from a measuring tube? Not to mention the nice nurses and stickers. I had no idea why Freddie would have cried. At my checkup the following week, I asked Dr. Depough,

"When can I get my shot? Can we do it today?"

He and the staff were surprised, but acquiesced and administered the vaccine ahead of schedule. I watched the needle pierce my skin, fascinated.

My parents also played a role in my interest in medicine.

My mom was an opera singer. When she wasn't rehearsing or performing, she was raising my brother and me and completing all the traditional female role tasks at home. And when she wasn't doing those things, she worked full time as the secretary of my school, Strasburg Elementary. The school employed a nurse named Thelma, who was lovely and kind and smelled like a vanilla candle. But she had many small town schools like ours to visit, so she was only in Strasburg Elementary once a month. The kids with day-to-day complaints — tummy aches, bruised knees and splinters — still came to the nurse's office every day, so my mom took up the role as acting nurse.

School was out at 3:30 each day. After the bell rang, I walked the short hallway to the front office where my mom was working. I played with the Paint program on an Apple computer and worked on my homework while she finished her paperwork. I helped staple, three-hole punch and file. And the best part — I learned about the day's illnesses and injuries. My mom took care of Cammie Smith when she fell off the monkey bars; John Klinger when he threw up in the school hallway; Kelsey Thompson when she peed in her chair; Stephanie Kelso when her pants ripped in front of the whole class; Tyler Swanson when he beat his head against a brick wall. I heard how she handled these miniature emergencies, and the stories served as my first lessons in basic medical care.

My parents bought me a children's book of anatomy. It contained a series of cartoons of a generic human outline, with each major body system represented. The circulatory system was a heart blob with red and blue tubes of varying sizes. The gastrointestinal system had squishier-looking brown, beige and red hoses from the mouth to the vertex between the legs. The nervous system was painted in cream and pink tones, with a ball of yarn in the head and hundreds of strings coming down, weaving into the arms, legs, fingers and toes. I studied these and then asked my mom which system I had.

"You have them all! We all have them all," she said.

"But how do they all fit?"

That one was tougher to explain.

As for my dad, he was a businessman and a good provider. If becoming a doctor is building a house, my dad supplied much of the bricks and mortar. He paid education expenses not covered by scholarships, for which I am very grateful. He still always ends each conversation with, "Let us know if you need anything."

I was always fascinated by human behavior and rare medical conditions. I watched "ER" every week and the Discovery Health Channel every night. In high school, I even convinced my parents to take me to hospitals and medical schools for spring vacations.

All of these things contributed to my idea of becoming a doctor. I knew it would be the most fulfilling, uplifting experience I could undertake. I was planning on doing my part to save the world.

FIRST WARNING SIGN

Over the summer before college, I volunteered five days a week at a cancer center. I drove the half hour each day to Anschutz Cancer Pavilion in a suburb of Denver. I restocked graham crackers and juice in waiting rooms and reorganized crinkled magazines in their metal racks. I mingled with other volunteers – mostly good-hearted, retired adults. I also attempted to interact with as many *medical people* as possible. One afternoon, I got lucky. A doctor there — a pathologist — brought me to his lab. He introduced me to the staff and showed me a few slides of tissue samples under a microscope. At the end of the day, he asked cautiously why I was volunteering.

"I want to be a doctor," I said.

His eyes flickered, changing from jovial to stern.

"I thought that might be the case," he said, "and that's why I wanted to talk to you. Have you thought a lot about this? Why do you want to be a doctor?"

I was surprised by his serious tone. I was accustomed to people instantly approving my goal and wishing me well. Their comments were usually whimsical, excited or, at worst, a little jealous. This was different. He looked like he was preparing to talk me out of my dream, so I became defensive.

"Yes, I have thought a lot about it. I have wanted to be a doctor since I was 4," I stated loudly. I explained my interest in anatomy and rattled off a few other details I thought would pull him back to my side.

He looked at me with sincerity, as if he were about to reveal a secret. He put his hand on my arm and said, "You have to read The House of God. Before you apply to medical school. Promise me."

I looked at him quizzically, trying to determine his motive. He seemed so insistent, so sure. Was he sorry he had become a doctor? Or did he think I wasn't up to the task?

"Okay, I promise."

He wasn't convinced.

"Really, I'll read it," I said.

At the end of the week, I purchased the book and read it. Interestingly, it didn't discourage me from applying to medical school at all. It intrigued me. I wanted to belong to this secret medical club.

LEARNING A VALUABLE SECRET

In June of 2002, just after my freshman year at Colorado State University, I was at a party in my college pad's backyard. I was 18 years old and desperate for information about how to get into medical school. My entire existence hinged on *getting into med school*.

It was getting dark. Word got to me – someone at the party had just been accepted to the University of Colorado Medical School. My heart began to race. I had a new mentor. I spent the next few minutes slyly making my way over to him.

He had sandy hair and was handsome with a slight build. He looked young but rugged and wore tough canvas pants. I couldn't help myself.

"So, how'd you get in?" I asked unabashedly.

He rolled his eyes a little. He smiled and took a long drink from a red plastic cup of beer. The suspense was killing me.

"I didn't really want to get in. Maybe that's the secret," he said.

My brain could not compute these sentences.

"But how do I get in? What do I do?" I pleaded.

"Listen, I was planning to do construction or go sail around the world for a year," he said. "I just sent an application and got in."

"But what was your GPA? What was on your resume?" I demanded. I was frantic, since this might be my only opportunity to talk to someone just accepted...into...med...school.

"They want to know you're a person," he said. "They can see straight through resume building." My eyes widened. I was receiving coveted information. My brain began scheming.

"Okay, so I need to show them I'm a person — should I add outside interests or hobbies?"

My imaginary mentor began to lose his patience with his imaginary pupil.

"No — that's not the poi...never mind. I'm gonna go grab another beer. Good luck, Frances."

And that was the end of my mentorship. I never saw him again.

Preparing my resume for medical school, I felt like I was weaving through a maze, collecting as many titles and experiences as possible.

1. I volunteered for and participated in charity events at every opportunity. I started an event called Bald 4 Bucks 4 Cancer, shaving my head and my friends' heads in support of cancer awareness (I donated the money to Anschutz, where I had volunteered). I joined Premedica, a group at Colorado State University that helps students prepare for medical careers. I led the Half-Day with a Doctor experience for fellow pre-med students. I participated in secular volunteer trips to Seattle, Chicago and Washington, D.C., partnering with health-based organizations (I helped raise money, cleaned parking lots, painted rooms, played with kids and handed out condoms).

2. I kept my grades up, but not perfect. I graduated with a 3.48 GPA in the honors department with a degree in philosophy, just shy of the 3.5 mark to graduate officially "With Honors." The philosophy courses taught me to read challenging material (which proved later to be an invaluable skill in medicine) and to think and write on a more professional level.

3. I remembered to have fun and showed it on paper. After my conversation with the party mentor, I realized that my college years were going to be my best bet at a carefree time. If I did land a slot in a medical school, I knew my social life would dwindle. I worked at a pizza shop. I partied (not on resume). I joined theater groups and eventually became the director of our student health center's theater group. My best friend Kat and I staged <u>The Vagina Monologues</u>.

I learned a great deal and became a stronger, more thoughtful person through the process of becoming a presentable medical school applicant. I joined every group I could, to experience something new — and to put it on my resume.

GETTING INTO MED SCHOOL

In the six months after college graduation, I was floating. I held a few temp jobs. Otherwise, I was consumed with sending applications to medical schools. My friend John (my college drinking/thinking buddy who also wanted to become a physician) and I worked as a team to get through the process. We frequented local bars and diners together planning our strategy and took an MCAT Review Course (the test to apply for entrance to med school) together.

At that time, the brightest spot in my life was my newly found partner, Judith Avers. I call her Jude.

We met at a festival in 2004 called Pride in the Park in Fort Collins, Colorado. She was playing her beautiful music on a big black guitar, and I fell shamelessly for her. Once we were together, she and I rented a Victorian style apartment and played grown-up. She worked as an aide to disabled clients in the blue-collar town of Greeley, Colorado, and I survived on my parents' kindness (money). But during most of this period, as I said, I held the part-time position of applying to med school. I sent secondary applications[1], waited to hear from schools about interviews, checked out and read books from the local library about HMOs and the current state of health care (to

---

[1] After the tedious first applications are sent to medical schools, applicants are sorted into a "no" pile and a "maybe" pile. Those in the "maybe" pile are invited to send a series of essays and another fee. These are called the "secondaries."

look smart in the upcoming interviews), and talked with John about what med school might be like and what we would do if we didn't get in. I slowly became nuttier and nuttier, waiting to see what the future held. I secretly began looking into becoming an American Sign Language interpreter. I had very little in the way of a backup plan. I sat on the porch every morning, literally waiting for the mail carrier.

Day after day.

I became despondent. A few rejection letters trailed in.

One evening, I drove to John's house to hang out. I spied an overstuffed envelope from Michigan State University College of Osteopathic Medicine on his dresser. I held it up. He looked at me with a red face.

"Yeah…so…I got an interview."

My heart sank. I knew that it meant I wouldn't be getting into this school, one of my last hopes.

"That's…great! Congratulations."

I slinked home, heartbroken. John had been too kind to tell me he had landed an interview first. It was a very real possibility that I would have to choose another career. I came home and sullenly notified Jude of the events of the day, and crawled into bed.

The next week, I received an overstuffed envelope from West Virginia School of Osteopathic Medicine, a.k.a. WVSOM, in Lewisburg, West Virginia. I had an interview. I was elated.

The interview led to my eventual acceptance.

I was now a bona fide med student.

MEDICAL SCHOOL

YEARS ONE AND TWO

Medical school is four years of intense learning sandwiched between undergraduate school and residency. Two of those years are in a classroom, and the other two are clinical, similar to an apprenticeship.

When I attended WVSOM 2005-2010, the med students were split into two pods: 85% of us in Systems Based Learning (SBL) and 15% of us in Problem Based Learning (PBL). SBL is the traditional med school model; these students attend eight hours of lectures a day and take scheduled exams. The curriculum is very structured.

I was a PBL student.

PBL is a method of learning medicine through cases, independent study and focused discussion groups. Instead of attending class eight hours a day, I had class sometimes as little as two hours a day. My small group of eight students would open a "case" of a fictitious patient, and have discussions based on that case. Most of our time was spent in independent study (our living rooms).

Over the course of those first two years, many subjects must be thoroughly covered: basic procedures, biochemistry, EKG reading, embryology, epidemiology, genetics, gross anatomy, histology, immunology, medical terminology, microbiology, neurobiology, osteopathic manipulative medicine (a.k.a. OMM), pathology, pharmacology, physiology and psychology.

The first year, I worked through medical knowledge wormholes, mostly using one of my textbooks, <u>Robbins and Cotran Pathologic Basis of Disease</u>, alternating frequently with <u>Stedman's Medical Dictionary</u>. We read voraciously, and then reconvened with our eight-person group and talked about what we had each learned. Eventually, we hit all the big targets: the coagulation cascade (how scabs form); the inflammation cascade (what happens after you hit your thumb with a hammer); digestion and enterohepatic circulation (the process of the body metabolizing drugs and food), etc.

Second year was similar but also entailed standardized patients (paid actors, pretending to be patients, so we could practice communication/examination skills), EKG reading and neuroanatomy. We also focused on pharmacology and specialties.

It was an overwhelming amount of information to absorb, but I didn't mind. I ate it up.

Gross anatomy was the class that left the biggest impression on me. We spent August through March working with cadavers, for four hours at a time, three days a week. We worked meticulously in groups of four, hovering over the bodies, matching up pink and gray formalin-laden 3D body parts with drawings/descriptions from our anatomy books.

I learned the following:

1. Always apply hand lotion, then two pairs of latex gloves. This prevents your hands from smelling bad all day.

2. Always insert scissors *closed* under the skin, then open to dissect the superficial tissues. This prevents injury to important structures.

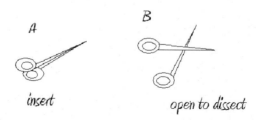

3. Wear an undershirt to stay warm in the cool lab. This tip also came in handy later in cold operating rooms.

4. Do as much work as you can while you are there.

5. Be efficient – find a balance between speed and patience.

6. Use mnemonics as much as possible. For instance, three nerves — L2, L3 and L4 — help men maintain an erection. How did we remember this, you might ask? "*L2, 3, 4 keeps the penis off the floor.*" Tricks such as these helped us learn many important but hard-to-remember details.

7. Know the complete anatomy of the azygos vein (a large blood vessel that runs longitudinally in the chest). Dr. Chapman, the chief anatomist, loves to ask about this vein (tip for the practical exam).

8. Memorize the cranial nerves and their respective foramen (holes in the skull). Dr. Mumford, assistant anatomist, loves to ask about them. Know these like states and capitals.

9. Use <u>Netter's Atlas of Human Anatomy</u>, AND photo-graphic anatomy books for better accuracy.

10. Don't bring Jude to gross anatomy lab (later revised to don't bring Jude to an OR, ER, or anywhere there might be thin plastic tubes, bodily fluids, hospital gowns or beeping machines).

Through gross anatomy class, I learned how it was possible to have all those systems crammed into one body. It was overwhelming and amazing. Taking apart a human is not like taking apart a machine. It is much more intricate, like trying to unravel an ecosystem. Everything is tied to everything else.

Think about the knee. The knee bone is connected to the thigh bone, yes. But there are also nerves, ligaments, muscles, tendons, lymphatics, menisci and fascia to contend with at every turn. There is the tissue level, the cellular level, the molecular level...so many layers of complexity. And that's the *simplest* large joint. There are hundreds of thousands of tiny networks working together just to bend and extend that single joint.

We dissected the cadavers in sections, for practical reasons: back, thorax, abdomen, upper extremity, lower extremity, pelvis, and lastly, head/neck.

The pelvis was the most complex area, a maze of organs, muscles and ligaments crisscrossing one another. I could never create a true mental map. The most memorable muscle of the pelvis: the iliopsoas — a muscle that traverses from the low back bones, attaches to the pelvic brim, and finally dives to hook onto the thigh bones. Lecturing with a PowerPoint presentation illustrating the intricacies of the pelvis, Dr. Mumford the anatomist stopped to marvel at it.

"What does it remind you of?" he asked, his head tilted, studying part of this muscle that begins at the pelvis like hair at the peak of a woman's forehead, draping down the head, over the neck and shoulders...

"A waterfall," he said. "That's what it reminds me of. Look at it cascading down from the pelvis to the femur."

Interesting.

I was also taken by the power and necessity of the abdominal diaphragm. It is the body's biggest and most multitalented pump. It separates the majority of the gastrointestinal system from the majority of the respiratory and circulatory systems. It pulls air into the lungs and gives the heart room to expand. It keeps the liver/spleen/pancreas from getting congested with old blood, stimulates the intestines to move, and keeps the stomach contents from regurgitating.

In times of stress, the diaphragm clenches in some areas and becomes flaccid in others. It changes from an efficient muscular piston to a cramping, irregularly-motioned flap of tissue. An anxious or distressed person will experience difficulties taking deep breaths, irregular heartbeats, constipation and/or diarrhea, abdominal pain, and reflux of food/acid from stomach into esophagus.

These are familiar symptoms for medical students and residents.

The beginning of my brain reprogramming was the other notable experience during those first med school years.

I noticed it in small ways. I would misplace my wallet. Or space out during conversation. Or couldn't quite keep up with a movie plot.

Then, it picked up speed. Jude and my other family began to accept and joke that I was getting brain-fried.

"Does she EVER know where her keys are?" they would laugh.

Often, I would suddenly reawaken mentally to find myself being stared at, usually by Jude.

"Did you hear me, babe?"

"Hm?"

"I just asked if you took a shower, already."

"Hm," I would say. I had spaced out during the conversation. And, I couldn't remember if I had indeed taken a shower or not.

Did I? Hm.

I felt my hair. It felt a little greasy.

"No, I didn't."

Friends gathered for a party at our house one evening during second year. Their names took a few more seconds to summons from my memory.

"Hey, Darron! How are you?"

"I'm good, France! Just back from Florida. Jane and I had a blast. We swam with dolphins and manatees..." he would keep talking, but my attention simply could not latch onto his words. Eventually, I found myself being stared at again.

"Frances? Where is your bathroom?"

"Oh, it's, um, just down the hall, and..." I would motion with my hand, instead of finding the words. Words were so hard to wrangle.

Med school buddies agreed with me. They felt like they were being robotized, that their brains were being mechanically reorganized to hold an ocean of medical facts. They also had a hard time particularly with attention and participating in rapid dialogue, especially if there were other distractions in the room.

Certain parts of the brain just had to shut down to make room.

FIRST SET OF BOARDS

From Day One of medical school, we were warned about the ominous-sounding "Boards" that loomed at the end of the second year. The Boards (a.k.a. COMLEX for D.O.s, and USMLE for M.D.s) would be the first in a lifelong string of national eight-hour exams to determine whether we knew enough to be called "Doctor." To me, the Boards sounded more like corporal punishment — as if we were going to be forced to run a gauntlet down a long corridor and be whacked repeatedly on our butts with two-by-fours. We knew that the Boards mattered — that we would flunk out of medical school if we didn't pass this one single exam, even if we had earned perfect grades for two years. Professors and doctors who taught us during years one and two always had the Boards to threaten us with if we got too cocky. We could each cite a few examples of med students who had failed their Boards; for them, it meant suddenly being shunned from doctorhood. They were now saddled with hundreds of thousands of dollars of debt and no training for any other job. The Boards were always on our minds.

To celebrate the end of second year of med school, Jude and I decided it would be nice to have a little vacation before I started my hardcore studying for the Boards. So, we rented a beach house with our friends Edith and Bobbi.

But for me the beach trip was anything but relaxing. All I could think was *"The Boards are a month away. Should I be studying now? Or should I relax?"* This mantra repeated in my mind throughout the vacation. I studied in the car, on the beach, on the way back from the beach, on long walks in the forest, etc.

When we returned home, I studied as hard as I could from 6 AM to 10 PM every day for three straight weeks. Jude and I studied together as a way to maintain communication. We held a constant banter of medical trivia. By the time The Day Before the Boards rolled around, Jude was spent. Even seeing her so drained, I could not exit the world of mnemonics and medical facts. I kept handing her my review books, begging her to ask me more questions. This all came to a fairly abrupt stop when we remembered a recent graduate's advice:

"When The Day Before the Boards comes, DON'T study. Just empty your brain and relax."

The Boards would be held in Charleston, West Virginia, more than an hour away from our home. We arrived the night before the Boards, and checked into a small hotel. Then, we padded down to the first-floor indoor swimming pool, and waded in. We softly pulled each other around by our hair on the surface of the water (Very calming. Try it sometime.).

We settled into our room and ordered pizza delivery. As soon as I took a bite, I started to tremble. My lips puffed up. Tears welled up and fell in two salty streams. All my pent-up emotions came out in a chaotic hurricane. I wept and wept into the pizza, marking the end of my Board studying marathon.

We slept soundly in the fluffiest white bed I had ever touched.

The next morning, I took the Boards. The exam took eight hours, with a lunch break (a Subway sandwich eaten with Jude on a curb outside the testing center).

I fretted for the next month, and then I got a letter.

I passed.

YEARS THREE AND FOUR

The clinical years (three and four) are in clinics and hospitals. I was stationed for much of this time in Weirton, West Virginia. My time was arranged in a series of four-week blocks called "rotations." In each rotation, I worked one-on-one with a variety of physicians who were experts in a range of specialties. Some of these were required, and some were elective. Here is the list of my rotations for those interested:

TWO WEEK ROTATIONS: addiction medicine, dermatology, otolaryngology (ENT), endocrinology, ophthalmology, plastic surgery, radiology, and urgent care.

FOUR WEEK ROTATIONS: cardiology, emergency medicine, general surgery, obstetrics/gynecology and psychiatry.

I also had eight weeks of pediatrics, twelve weeks of internal medicine and a whopping *sixteen* weeks of family medicine.

Because I was lucky enough to have a few savvy attendings throughout my rotations (mostly Dr. Makar), I also spent a single day with an attending of each of the following specialties: anesthesiology; cardiac surgery; gastroenterology; neurology; podiatry; pulmonology; rheumatology and urology. WVSOM provided some basic objectives for each rotation. For a few of the rotations, we had an examination or computer module to complete in addition to the clinical experience.

These years were fragmented. Each rotation was just long enough to get to know that doctor's office, personality and quirks, then say goodbye. The curriculum was not uniform. Each physician I worked with taught me small lessons, but each instructor had no idea what I had learned from the previous one. This led to a colorful, disjointed tour through the clinical medical world.

One internist drove me around in his Smart Car and taught me a diagnostic approach to liver diseases. A family medicine doc quizzed me daily on various topics, introduced me to his family and took Jude and me out to Pizza Hut. An OB/GYN took me out for breakfast after we delivered a baby together at Weirton Medical Center. It was two years of seemingly random experiences with doctors, generously teaching me what they knew.

GRADUATION

I woke up at 4:30 AM with a vertiginous hangover: too much celebrating the night before. I walked to the bathroom sink and cupped my hand under lukewarm silky water, gulping as much as I could hold in my stomach. I stumbled back to bed, and the next thing I heard was my 7 AM alarm. I dressed and quickly drove down to WVSOM to find my family some good seats for the outdoor ceremony, only to discover that Jude had graciously already done so.

I knew this would be a wonderful day, but I was mostly looking forward to the following weekend; Jude and I were getting married! Although this would not be a legal ceremony (West Virginia had not yet legalized same-sex marriage), it would be a wedding — complete with dresses, families and friends, rings, vows and wedding cake.

Graduation day was hot and humid, and my family suffered through it to the bitter end, since alphabetically my last name is pretty late in the show. After the ceremony, I was greeted with smiles, hugs and lots of picture taking.

Jude and I shared the good news with our family and friends: I had landed a three-year position as a resident at UPMC Shadyside, a hospital in Pittsburgh, in the family medicine residency program. I had chosen family medicine because it combines the areas of medicine I love: psychiatry, pediatrics, gynecology, internal medicine, musculoskeletal medicine (aches and pains) and geriatrics.

Remarks from well-wishers were mostly happy and hopeful, though some warned of difficulties ahead.

"You made it, babe!"

"These upcoming years are going to be amazing, but incredibly arduous."

"Please know how happy and proud we are of you. We love you."

"You two are getting married next week? What are you thinking?"

"Congratulations."

After the graduation ceremony, I bumped into Dr. Light and Dr. Schumacher, two of my advisers. Dr. Light told me I was beginning "the most rewarding part of my life," then smiled and walked off looking for cookies and punch. In response to that comment, Dr. Schumacher furrowed his brow and said, "I don't think 'the most rewarding part of your life' is the most accurate depiction of what's about to happen to you. It's rewarding, eventually. But it is really, really tough. Actually, it's horrible."

Dr. Schumacher handed me a small pile of polished stones in a pouch and explained they were to be used to ponder and to calm myself down in residency. After learning of our upcoming wedding, his wife cornered Jude and I and scolded us for getting married, spouting very high statistics (80%) for divorce during residency (I later searched but could find no basis for such a statistic.).

At my party there were thoughtful presents (Snoopy dressed as a doctor, fancy pens...), and lots of alcohol. Dr. Redding (another one of my wonderful advisers) fell asleep in her chair from exhaustion and too much champagne. I had an enormous sense of relief, joy and anticipation. It felt like walking into a blooming garden after a long winter. Jude and I knew what was to come with my residency — hard work and fun and enjoying life in a city (we would be moving to Pittsburgh, a real city!). We were excited about this new chapter in our lives, and we chose to ignore the few naysayers.

Jude and I were married the next weekend and had a ball. Our friends and family trekked in from far and wide for the occasion, but most of our guests were from Lewisburg, where WVSOM is located. The ceremony was officiated by Peg and Hermes, our surrogate parents in medical school. It was the best wedding I have ever attended, and many people said so too. Thank god we did it. My ring later helped me through some tough moments, and I suspect I would be single and unhappy today had we not committed to the long haul together before it started. We wouldn't know it until later, but Dr. Schumacher's wife's negative comment helped spur us on as a team through the most challenging times.

RESIDENCY

"THE MATCH"

In the course of residency, which generally lasts three to five years, medical school graduates receive training in a specialty – family medicine or emergency medicine or surgery, etc. The location of that residency is determined by a process called "The Match" (or NRMP, National Resident Matching Program), a placement service that uses algorithms to match fourth-year medical students with their rank-order list of hospitals. It's similar to Rush (that is, the process of getting into a sorority or fraternity in college). It's also like the military; you go where The Match sends you, and that's that. There is no going back.

To finalize a successful placement through The Match, fourth-year medical students and residency programs all across the country "court" one another. The courting occurs via "audition rotations," interviews and clinical experiences during the third and fourth years of medical school. Each side tries to get a sense of the other's strengths and weaknesses. Then the students rank the programs:

"Hmmm....let's see...Johns Hopkins No. 1, and Harvard No. 2..."

While the programs rank the students:
"Hmmm...that med student is a cousin of one of our current residents...let's rank him in our top 10..."

Each side then submits their respective list (the med students must pay a fee). Months later, out pops the "Match List"—which is golden because it dictates who goes where. Now the new first-year residents — called interns — know where they are going to live and work for the next several years, and residency directors know who they will be training. Celebration ensues for many. But for those who do not get a Match, there is a Scramble list (unfilled, unwanted spots…yes, that's the real term). These unfortunate un-Matched med students have 48 hours to call the programs on the Scramble list, and they often end up in places they do not belong, even in *specialties* they did not want.

After applying to ten residency programs across the country, I received interview offers from all ten choices. This was a much different process than applying to medical school, where I had landed a *single* interview from ten secondaries. I chose to interview at seven programs. After those interviews (big expense, driving/flying all over the country for these), I whittled the list down to three programs for my Match rank list:

1. UPMC Shadyside Family Medicine Residency Program in Pittsburgh, PA

2. UMASS Family Medicine in Fitchburg, Massachusetts

3. Sisters of Charity Family Medicine in Buffalo, New York

My friend John and I both Matched our first choices, which happened to be in the same city. We would work in neighboring hospitals — me at Shadyside, John at UPMC St. Margaret's. Jude and I moved into an apartment with our cats. John and his partner, Matt, bought a house nearby, about 30 minutes away. John was like my male mirror. We would continue the journey toward doctorhood together.

ORIENTATION WEEK

Orientation Week (an immediate prelude to residency) is packed. Interns meet fellow interns; review key medical procedures (*or are exposed to them for the first time*); explore the new city; learn the layout of the various hospitals in which they will be working; read and sign lots of paperwork (*"sign here, and here, and here, and here..."*); take down important phone numbers (*"here's the number to call when you are worried about a lawsuit, and here's the number for our confidential counseling group in case you become suicidal..."*); and learn hospital logistics (*we learned four distinct computerized Electronic Health Records systems, complete with dictation codes, passwords and instructions for each*).

The first three days of Orientation Week at Shadyside Hospital were the most interesting.

Day 1: That first morning at Shadyside Hospital, there were eight of us shiny, green, brand-new family medicine interns. Some of us were M.D.s, some D.O.s. Some were from the United States, and some were not. Residents from med schools outside the U.S. are called foreign or international medical grads (FMGs, or IMGs), and most of them were practicing physicians in their home countries. However, in order to become practicing physicians in the U.S., all foreign doctors (regardless of specialty or level of training) must complete a U.S. residency program.

On our first meeting, I tried my best to remember my fellow interns:

1. **Akira.** Thin, thoughtful, very polite, married, from Japan. He was a practicing physician for about a decade prior to matriculation to the U.S.

2. **Nikki.** A single, petite blonde from Canada who never stopped giggling. She was bright and witty and had the best penmanship of the group.

3. **Heath.** Large, beefy all-American from Montana, married, proud of his new truck, planning to practice full-spectrum family medicine in the boonies.

4. **Tomoko.** Even-keeled, friendly, engaged to her long-distance boyfriend, Vince, in California. She grew up in both the U.S. and Japan, and is truly the most bi-cultural person I have ever known.

5. **Angela.** The quintessential Type A personality from the Midwest. Single. She was the one who wrote down all of our birthdays during Orientation Week.

6. **Sara.** Married to Jojo (below), another intern. This couple from India were very bright, friendly, positive and professional at every turn. Sara was diligent and never complained.

7. **Jojo.** Married to Sara (above). He was quiet, laid-back, always with a smile, easy to be around.

8. **Frances.** Eager to learn, from Small Town America. She has wanted this moment forever.

Day 2: We were given our schedules for the year. Debbie Philips and Susan Worthers, who were office managers and organizers of Orientation Week, handed them out. Each schedule was divided into 13 periods (rotations) for the year, similar to how I was accustomed to living for the past two years of medical school.

After handing out the schedules, Debbie and Susan walked cautiously over to me. Debbie said, "Frances, it looks like you got the tough schedule this year. There is one every year. You have a bad string of rotations right at the beginning: Floors, Children's, Magee Womens, Floors, Nursery."

I looked at her blankly. I didn't understand.

"We tried to make accommodations for everyone's requests, but sometimes things like this happen. But we can try to change it…"

"Oh, I'll be fine!" I said. "I'm excited to get started. Thanks for looking over the schedules."

Debbie and Susan exchanged a worried look that I chose to ignore.

"You're sure you'll be okay? If you want to change it, today's the only day to make an alteration. After that, you're locked in."

"It's fine. It's great! Don't worry about it," I said.

What difference did it make, I wondered, to have a small string of tougher rotations clustered together or scattered throughout the year? This is what I had come for — to get training.

"*Bring it on*," I thought.

"Now that you all have your schedules," Susan explained, "it is time to get coverage for your vacation time."

Hmm?

We all looked at each other.

Now? We need to know our vacation dates for the entire year?

"Yes, you need to organize vacation for the entire year," Susan said. "Right now."

We scrambled. We began bartering with one another, flipping through our calendars, texting our spouses and mothers, and sweet-talking one another as best we could.

"Oh! One more thing," they said. "There are a few 'mandatory months' during which you are not permitted to take vacation time. All rotations in bold-face are off limits. Regarding vacation on your community medicine rotation, you must agree with your fellow interns about which days you will take off." We scrambled again. I looked at my schedule — of the 13 periods, nine were in bold face.

Okay, so there would be four possible months to take my 15 vacation days, with a few stipulations. We were slightly confused, but continued following orders, bargaining with one another for the best vacation slots. We texted our families to tell them we would not be home for Thanksgiving, Christmas, Easter…

That evening, we were warmly welcomed by all the faculty and residents. A graduation celebration for the third-year residents ensued, with skits, music and slide shows of all the graduating residents. We learned about their histories and saw them proudly hold their residency diplomas high. I was impressed by their camaraderie. Afterward, there was a welcome party at the program director's home, complete with local microbrews and organic produce. Jude was encouraged to participate. We felt quite at home.

Day 3: This was procedure review day. In the morning, all eight of us took a bus across town to a training site to practice placing central lines (large-bore IVs that are inserted into the veins in the neck and groin) into dummies. We inserted our needles into the large plastic veins. If we pulled back red Kool-Aid (our substitute for fake blood) into the syringe, we nailed it. This was my third time working on central lines.

The afternoon was women's care review with standardized patients. Translation: We practiced doing Pap smears on women who were monetarily compensated for allowing interns to insert speculums into their vaginas. This was not a worry for me; I had performed many pelvic examinations in medical school. We were briefly instructed on the use of the specula and how to talk through the exam with the patient. We were then split into three groups; each group had at least one intern, an attending physician and a standardized patient. My group: Akira, Dr. Longfellow (our attending), Sherrice (our standardized patient) and me. I went first, slipping the speculum in easily, talking the patient through the procedure.

Then, I watched as Akira performed his very first pelvic examination. He had been a physician in Japan, but he had not received gynecologic training; he had been an E.R. doctor, not a family medicine doctor. It was like watching a one-armed man tie a shoelace or peel an egg. I wanted to save him, but this was a moment he had to work through on his own.

"Sorry. Sorry. Oh, so, so sorry," he sputtered in his soft accent, as sweat beaded on his forehead and ran down his face. He got through it after about 15 slow minutes, with Dr. Longfellow patiently guiding him through the procedure.

That evening was the capstone of procedure day: cardio-pulmonary resuscitation (CPR), basic life support (BLS) and advanced life support (ACLS) retraining. I walked by Akira and watched as he expertly intubated (inserted a breathing tube through the mouth and into the trachea) his dummy in three seconds flat. His skills as an emergency medicine doctor for 10 years shined brightly.

We each had our weaknesses and our strengths.

FIRST ROTATION

"Heart Station" (reading EKGs and helping with cardiac stress tests) was my opening rotation of intern year, which started immediately after Orientation Week. Every day I carried a small red notebook in which I wrote everything I learned throughout the day...uh, I mean...morning. We were generally done around noon. I spent the rest of each day studying and spending time with Jude.

This rotation was two weeks of only slight awkwardness, working with a different cardiology attending every day. EKG reading was luckily a skill I already had under my belt, thanks to a Polish physician I had worked with on a rural rotation in my fourth year of medical school. He had "graded" my EKGs daily, creating one of my most valuable learning experiences.

The second day on Heart Station, the senior resident on Floors paged me. She assigned me a patient to see in the hospital. He was a young male with acute abdominal pain. An hour before Heart Station rotation each morning, I visited, evaluated and ordered medications and bloodwork for (also known as "rounding") the patient, and then completed the morning of EKGs and stress tests.

The third day, after seeing my patient and writing orders for him in the morning and reading my EKGs, I asked Jude to lunch. We skipped merrily to a fine Italian restaurant near the hospital. I brazenly ordered a glass of red wine. This was going great. Dr. Schumacher had it all wrong.

During Heart Station, the most helpful information I learned (apart from the differences and indications for various stress tests) was which cardiologists were the most intern-friendly. I discovered which doctors were open to being paged with questions and those who didn't mind being consulted late on a Friday afternoon. I learned which doctors had a softer approach, and which ones were more interested in procedures.

All in all, it was the easiest rotation I ever had, including medical school.

At least three attendings in my time at Heart Station, upon learning that I was an intern, said in a soothing tone, "It gets better. Hang in there."

My internal response to this was, "Hang in there? I'm here because I want to be here. I don't need that advice. This is a piece of cake!"

But in the back of my mind I couldn't help but wonder — would I need that advice?

"CALL"

Doctors work through the day, then sometimes work through the night. The night work is called being "on call." Residents are on call a lot. Usually, this means staying in the hospital all night long. As an intern, with a few exceptions, I had a more experienced "senior resident" (second- or third-year resident) on call with me who supervised. My first year, I took call 88 times. Second year, I was on call about one day per week. And third year was best of all; I worked 11 total weekends, and never had to be physically in the hospital at night.

The mood and level of intensity of the evening on call depended upon:

1. Who I was on call with, and

2. How busy the hospital was.

Nikki and I were always a perfect call pair. We giggled through every evening on call together like kids at a slumber party. Between admissions, we played YouTube videos for each other, laughed about the training process and told stories about our previous lives. Somehow, those nights with Nikki always seemed easier. We shared a white cloud (see below).

Residents are often superstitious about being on call. There are many rules and strange beliefs, sporadically followed in different programs. For example:

1. You must not mention the word 'admission'; it will bring on an admission.

2. You must sleep with the light on between admissions to prevent admissions.

3. Some residents are 'black clouds' and some are 'white clouds.' You always want to be on call with a 'white cloud' to avoid having a 'bad call night.'[2] You can do nothing to become a white cloud; you simply are, or you aren't.

4. You must never verbally acknowledge when it is quiet; it will bring on an admission or a disaster.

5. You must never mention the name of a patient; this will bring them into the Emergency Department.

6. Full moons bring on terrible or very strange call evenings.

7. You must never buy a newspaper or magazine if you are going to be on call; it will bring on disaster.

8. You must not read or watch television on call nights; you will get slammed with work.

Most hospitals have facilities where doctors on call can sleep, grab a snack or just find a quiet respite for a while, in the downtime between caring for patients. These are called call rooms. Call rooms vary from hospital to hospital — that is, some offer perks like showers, refreshments and TV, while others resemble a monk's cell. So I wanted to be prepared. When I was a med student, I read a blog that featured an article called "What to Bring Your First Night on Call." This concept appealed to the packrat/organizer side of me; I had been the type of kid who packed 10 days early for a trip. I thought about what I

---

2 A bad call night entails having many and/or difficult admissions, patients becoming critically ill in the hospital, losing one's stethoscope, etc.

might bring: a mini-fridge? Pajamas? A book? A laptop or DVD player? Medical school allowed me to sample a few call rooms to get a feel for the answers:

St. Margaret's (Pittsburgh, PA) — quite spare; contained bunk beds in a clean room.

St. Joseph's (Philadelphia, PA) — had a single bed, a variety of appliances (toaster oven, electric kettle), and an antiquated computer. It was quirky and lived-in, and held small treasures of previous tenants, such as an old cracked stethoscope and medical textbooks from the 1960s.

Good Samaritan (Corvallis, OR) — on the tour of this program, I wasn't shown any call rooms. I suspected this was because it was such a new residency; maybe none even existed.

Shadyside (Pittsburgh, PA) — three rooms at the end of a long hall of call rooms (many specialties had call rooms there). Each room had a single bed and a desk with a phone and a computer. The resident lounge was nearby.

For this superficial perk and many other reasons, I chose Shadyside, the hospital with the call room in close proximity to the resident lounge, which had free coffee and hot cocoa 24/7.

The best thing about Shadyside's call rooms: an up-to-date, working computer, all to myself. Otherwise, reality was a little different from what I had envisioned...

The hours I spent in call rooms were tense. At Shadyside, many nights on call during intern year were crammed. Page after page, every few minutes. I would lie down on top of the blanket with my shoes on and both pagers next to my left ear.

Some nights I had a little sleep, others I had none. The one thing I had to get used to was the hospital sheets, which smelled terrible. The odor was faint, but present – a mix of mucus, blood, diarrhea and cheap detergent. But I got used to the smell after the first year and started sleeping in them when I could.

I ate at the cafeteria (pizza, yogurt, chips, ice cream or, if it was slow, a baked potato) and stuffed my pockets with quick snacks (granola bars, chocolates, string cheese). I (along with the other residents) also knew the code to the patient nutrition supply room, so I had no shortage of saltines and ginger ale.

Call differed, from year to year.

First year: I was terrified, nauseated, constantly on edge. Frequently, I received multiple pages at once: 1-7888. 1-7291. 2-9928. (All of these are phone numbers around the hospital.) CONDITION C: 594-1 (this meant I had to hurry to room 594-1 and help with a suddenly critically ill patient). I scrambled to call each one back, as more pages poured in. I quickly learned to stick to a consistent system: Write the pages down in order. Delete the pages from pager. Get to a computer and phone as quickly as possible. Open the electronic medical record. Briskly call each number back, "This is family medicine, you paged?" Discuss the issue with the caller (usually my senior resident assigning me an admission or a nurse with a patient problem). Document my work on paper and electronically.

If it was my senior calling with a new admission, I would start an admission form and quickly check the patient's details in the electronic chart on my computer before heading down to the ED (Emergency Department) to see the patient. Then I would make a plan and discuss it with both the senior resident (in person) and the sleepy attending (over the phone), and finalize the orders and the admission note. The whole process of admitting a patient to the hospital, from the senior's page to the completion of the admission note took anywhere from one to five hours.

If the page was from a nurse, I would discuss with him or her how to care for the problem at hand. Can't sleep? Melatonin. Itchy? Benadryl. Fever? Need more information — the nurse may have to:

1. Do a blood/urine culture and chest X-ray or

2. If in process, stop a blood transfusion (this can cause fever) or the most common call-question answer:

3. Give 500mg of Tylenol.

Often, the pages required me to travel from one part of the hospital to another. There was drastic variance in types of pages. Sometimes the issues were minor – checking an order or changing a dose. But sometimes it was serious or, worse, sometimes the caller didn't know it was serious. So I had to have extremely keen listening skills. Headache in a patient could be linked to simple dehydration, but it could also mean a hemorrhagic stroke.

I spent about 70 percent of the night walking up and down hallways, examining and talking to patients, and answering pages; 20 percent of the night dictating my notes about these issues, and 10 percent of the night with palpitations waiting for the next problem to occur.

Needless to say, I didn't have time to figure out where to put a mini-fridge.

Second Year: I was more confident and had fewer pages. I completed half the admissions alone (much more efficiently than I had as an intern), and assigned the other half of the admissions to my intern. I also got a little more sleep and had a little less stress.

Third Year: When my pager would go off, I would get out of bed and call the number back. I would talk to the nervous med student or intern. Then, I would go back to sleep — it wasn't a great sleep, but I was home in my own bed. Ahhh.

Garb/Equipment

When on call as an intern, I wore the required blue scrubs, a long white coat and my own personal touch: a tool belt to carry all the equipment I thought I needed. The belt, which I had purchased at a hardware store, had a metal hook to hold a hammer. But the hook was too big for a reflex hammer. I tried to remove the hook, but it was no use — it was so securely in place, even wire cutters wouldn't budge it. I tried weaving my stethoscope into the hook a few times, but it was more trouble than it was worth. So I just wore my stethoscope around my neck like everyone else. The tool belt held my reflex hammer, otoscope, ophthalmoscope and a stack of papers and books explaining how to save people's lives. After the first three months, I shed the tool belt because it was too cumbersome. The hook kept hitting the backs of chairs and nurses. I also found out I didn't really need all those tools. Plus, I was trying to shed my "Bob the Builder" nickname.

As a senior resident (years two and three), I stretched the rules and wore khaki pants and a white T-shirt under a blue scrub top, topped with a fleecy brown hoodie. Body temps drop a bit between 1 AM and 5 AM, so the hoodie and T-shirt provided me with extra warmth during those odd hours. Even while I slept, I kept in my breast pocket the few materials I truly needed — patient information lists, phone numbers of attendings and hospital departments, and a copy of the <u>Maxwell Quick Medical Reference</u> guide. The only thing that wasn't attached to me was my stethoscope, often rendering me stethoscopeless after I clomped down to the ED after being awakened for an admission.

Third Year: Whatever I wanted to wear. Again – call was taken from home.

FLOORS AT SHADYSIDE

Floors was a long month, but I enjoyed it. We worked Floors four times a year, to gain experience taking care of hospitalized patients (and supply Shadyside Hospital with extremely cheap labor). The most rewarding part — I felt like I was a real doctor, taking care of real patients...because I was.

I did a lot of walking around the hospital, talking to people, thinking and reading, and typing. I learned so much. Each day was packed full of tedious little tasks, fixing things I had forgotten, interviewing patients and their families, answering pages, and writing notes and orders. It was the busy life of a hospital doctor.

Floors rotations were exciting and full of learning, but also very draining physically, emotionally and mentally, especially when I had a dying patient, a demanding patient family or an attending I didn't agree with. There was also stress at sign-in, when I was assigned a patient with a life-threatening infection or organ failure. But even a commonplace diagnosis like new-onset diabetes or pneumonia kept me on high alert. I was the one on patrol to make sure the patient didn't die.

During my intern year, the Floors schedule was too complex to explain, but I essentially worked 75-100 hours a week and officially logged 80 hours a week, to prevent my program from being flagged for work-hour violations. By the time I was a second year resident, the program had changed the Floors schedule to "7 A to 7 P," which meant 12-hour shifts, six days a week. What it did not take into account was the seven-minute review before sign-in of patient care from the overnight residents, the 40-minute sign-out, the 30- to 60-minute leftover dictated notes after sign-out. (Dictated notes: Every patient encounter requires documentation of what the patient said, what his/her examination showed and our assessment and course of action.) Those things added about two more hours. And the driving/parking/walking back and forth to car time added more time; now we have an additional three hours. So that meant I had 15 hours dedicated to work and nine hours for everything else (sleeping, showering, eating, living, etc.).

Here is how I fit it all in:

6:00 AM   Alarm

~ Press snooze 3 times ~

6:12 AM   Get out of bed

6:13 AM   Fix hair / Wash face

6:16 AM   Put bread in toaster

6:20 AM   Get dressed

6:21 AM   Feed cats

6:23 AM   Put butter/jam on toast

6:25 AM   Organize supplies (white coat, books, etc.)

6:28 AM   Kiss Jude goodbye

6:31 AM   Drive/eat toast

6:47 AM	Park in garage
6:51 AM	Walk up steps to Three East, our family medicine hangout / place to sign in
6:53 AM	Review overnight labs on the computer
7:00 AM	Sign-in

7 AM to 7 PM on Floors was semi-organized, pressured chaos. Each day I evaluated and treated six to 10 hospitalized patients; responded to dozens of pages; completed one to seven admissions; grabbed a quick lunch; had various meetings (with dying patients' families, advisers, our program director and with a group who worked on hospital quality improvement), responded to emails and patient phone messages (*"Can Dr. Southwick call me back? My legs are swelling but I can't come to the office..."*); taught med students; read up on all manner of medical problems; gave lunchtime lectures to my fellow residents; consulted with nurses, attendings, residents and specialists; put in orders for various patients (for example: check vital signs every eight hours, turn the oxygen down, change the Tylenol to ibuprofen, draw more blood in the morning); completed patient notes and dictations. To complete all this within my 12-hour shift, I shaved off unnecessary minutes and multitasked. For instance, I would teach a med student about heart failure while walking to a patient room; I'd respond to a page on the phone while looking up patient orders on the computer; I'd eat a snack while dictating a note. I texted while on the toilet. I always ate my breakfast while driving to the hospital. And I took my "alone time" while driving home, listening to Ani DiFranco or NPR.

Here is how my day ended:

7:00 PM	Sign-out begins
7:40 PM	Walk out of Three East
7:45 PM	Get into car
7:57 PM	Park in front of apartment
8:05 PM	Shower, put on pajamas
8:20 PM	Eat dinner and zone out
9:20 PM	Talk to Jude for a while: "How was your day?"
9:35 PM	Finish note dictations
10:30 PM	Fall asleep on couch
11:15 PM	Get awakened by Jude to go to bed
11:30 PM	Climb into bed
6:00 AM	Alarm

I allocated about 16 minutes per day for Jude. We had a date night once a week too, which meant my time for sleeping took a hit, and I had to be more efficient at work, but it was worth it. I had to limit date nights to a two-hour maximum so I could perform the next day.

Fortunately, we lived very close to the hospital, which meant I had a little extra time in my schedule (usually allocated to sleeping) in comparison with some of my cohorts. If I allocated eight hours for sleeping (too generous, but just for the sake of discussion), I had 44 minutes left for eating dinner, showering, fixing my hair, getting dressed/undressed, feeding cats, brushing teeth, walking to and from car, taking out trash, calling relatives...

I did have one day off per week, though. Fortunately for me, Jude was very considerate and handled most of the basic household chores (washing dishes, cleaning, shopping, cooking) during my work hours, so that on my days off we could go on a hike or to a movie or just cuddle. I also tended to sleep more on those days. I felt terrible for the residents who did not have a spouse to support them through that difficult time; some admitted they survived on ramen noodles and hospital food.

Akira and Heath each had wives. Nikki was in a relationship with another resident. Sara and Jojo quietly supported each other without a peep of complaint; their stoic journeys through residency are still a mystery to me. Tomoko's boyfriend, Vince, lived across the country, so they Skyped at the times they were both at home and awake (they also had the barrier of a time difference). And Angela remained single the whole time and ended up winning Best Resident of the Country at the end of third year. I guess she didn't need sleep: She was the fastest talker, typist and walker I have ever met. So that must have saved her a few minutes. She also saved those 16 minutes I spent with Jude.

THE BLUE-LIPPED LADY

One month as an intern on Floors, I was taking care of eight patients in the hospital. One woman was very sick, having on and off respiratory failure, and I was concerned about her. One morning I walked into her room to find that her lips had turned blue. She was sleepy but I was able to rouse her easily. She was on 6 liters of oxygen by nasal cannula (which means she had to be supplemented with a moderate amount of oxygen to breathe). I hurried out to the nurse's station and looked at her oxygen saturation (her body's oxygen level), which should have been 95-100 percent. Her monitor read 72 percent, which had sent an alarm blaring. Even so, no one looked flustered. I found an aide and called the respiratory technician to the room STAT.

Two respiratory techs rushed in, and we took another measurement of the oxygen saturation — it was now 75 percent. We cranked the oxygen up full blast, 15 liters. She turned pink, and her number shot up to 94 percent. I sighed with relief.

A nurse rushed in, demanding, "What the hell is going on here?"

I explained the blue lips, the low indications on the monitor and the increase in oxygen we had made.

"Those things," she said, pointing to the monitor, "Are always wrong! What is wrong with you? You paged someone STAT? Are you trying to give me a heart attack?"

I walked out of the room, inviting the nurse to come with me. I composed myself and attempted a civilized conversation with her. She was a skinny, bitter woman who reeked of cigarette smoke. I quickly assessed the situation – she was upset I had noticed something about a patient she was responsible for, and she resented it, especially since I was a fresh intern. I looked into her eyes and said, "Listen, we both want what's best for the patient. I did what I did for her safety."

"Well, what the hell were you thinking?" she snapped. "You can't page someone STAT unless there is an emergency!"

"It *was* an emergency," I said. "Her sats were dropping. She was getting confused, and her lips were cyanotic (blue)."

"Well, those monitors are always wrong! You got everyone on the floor in a panic!"

We went on like this for a few minutes. My heart rate began to climb, as I became angrier and angrier.

"Listen, you fucked up my relationship between me and my patient. It was an emergency and she is better. OK? I am going to get something to eat." I turned and left her in imaginary dust.

That was probably my most intense argument with a nurse (normally I got along very well with all staff, especially nurses), but my response signified a change in me: I was beginning to trust my instincts as a doctor. Plus it was a reminder to eat a morning snack.

I discussed the blue-lipped lady with my senior resident and my attending. They weren't concerned.

"You're really worried about her, aren't you?" the attending asked patronizingly.

"Yeah, she seems pretty sick."

"Don't you worry. She'll bounce back."

The next morning, I walked into an escalated version of the previous day's scene. The same patient again was blue around her mouth, and was unresponsive. I started to sweat. I called the respiratory team. They put a non-rebreather (oxygen mask) on her, which raised her saturation from 70 percent to 90 percent. She was now awake and terrified.

"We are working on getting your breathing back on track," I explained to her. I asked an aide to get a manual set of vital signs. Her blood pressure was 70/40, too low, which was a bad sign. I decided to page the ICU doctor (called an intensivist) for help.

Dr. Spook arrived in a floor-length white coat. He had a blond crewcut, a razor-sharp nose and cold, beady blue eyes.

"What's up?" he asked, seemingly bored.

I explained the situation. The patient needed a central line for a life-saving drug to be started. I had practiced inserting these (reference the red Kool-Aid), but wasn't confident enough to place a real one without supervision. Plus, the patient needed to be transferred to the ICU to receive the medicine, and that required an intensivist.

"You ever heard the phrase 'Your poor planning ain't my emergency'?" he said with a smirk.

I glowed inside with fury.

"She is tanking," I said. "Aren't you the intensivist? I'm the intern. I need your help."

I had never been so direct with a superior in my life. I don't know why, but my involvement with this patient seemed to be continually abutted against doubt, apathy and complacency. Dr. Spook eventually put in the line after finishing his coffee. The patient died in the ICU a few days later.

I later discussed my Dr. Spook encounter with Tomoko, who also had worked with him. Tomoko said that during her ICU rotation, Dr. Spook would round, coffee in hand, with a pack of young white coats, from 6 AM to 4 PM. He wouldn't stop until his legs began to cramp, and he would then do squats in the nurses' station while the residents waited, standing in the hall, starving and exhausted. On a daily basis he would push Tomoko to the point of defeat in front of her peers, asking her question after question until she finally didn't have an answer or was too flustered to speak (in the medical training world, this is universally called "pimping"). I guess he didn't like family medicine residents.

The next year, he moved out of state — the hospital shone brighter without him.

CHILDREN'S HOSPITAL FLOORS

Sign-in would be at 6 AM sharp. This moved my schedule up a bit, reference Floors chapter.

At 5:30 AM, I arrived at the hospital. I leapt out of my car, excited but also terrified to be in a brand-new location with a whole new set of regulations, policies and schedules. I hurried through a maze of buildings and hallways, asking a few people in uniform if they knew where I was supposed to be. Finally, I came upon a group of similarly bewildered newbies, waiting nervously for our computer training.

The instructor was late. We all half-acknowledged, half-ignored each other. Then I spotted a face that looked somewhat familiar. Could it be Nancy? Was it Nancy from med school, the Nancy I thought I was going to be in residency with?

It was. But she didn't look like the Nancy I had known before. She looked terrible.

"Oh my God, I didn't think I would see you again!" I said. "How are you? How is your program?"

She glared at me. After no small talk to break the ice, she told me she was struggling and now had to force herself to simply show up every day. She grumbled about her job duties, her hours, her patients, her attending physicians, and generally had nothing positive to say.

I was shocked. Nancy had been a positive, shining star in our class. She was known for her bright blonde hair, sparkling eyes, movie-star-white teeth and bubbly personality. Now her hair was flat and her cheeks were hollow. She was dressed in a faded sweatshirt over scrubs. She said she had just had a baby. She had not disclosed her pregnancy to any of the residency directors during her search before the Match, to prevent discrimination against her. She explained that instead of ranking Shadyside as No. 1 in the Match, she had chosen a suburban program with housing near the hospital, so her family life would be more stable.

She looked so beaten up, and I was worried about her.

I was also pretty worried about myself; about caring for hospitalized pediatric patients. Regrettably, I had somehow skirted our medical school's "mandatory" month of inpatient pediatrics. I had done this, I suppose, because I had a lack of experience dealing with children, let alone *sick* children, and I was intimidated. At the time, I had scoffed at the requirement, saying it was a waste of training for *every* med student to complete an inpatient pediatric rotation; that only "peds-interested" people should be doing those rotations. So, the administration let it slide.

I was always late for evening sign-in at Children's. I worked at Shadyside Family Health Center (our residency program's outpatient doctor's office) a few half-days through the week, seeing patients as a family doctor might, only with supervision. My office hours at the health center were from noon to at 5 PM. This meant that I worked in one area of the city, then ran out of the office, across the medical campus to my car, drove like a bat out of hell to the Children's parking lot, where I then sprinted the half mile from the parking lot to the nurses' station where all the Children's residents were waiting, annoyed that the family medicine resident was 20 minutes late…again.

Call nights at Children's involved walking around the hospital and checking on kids, making sure orders were right and doing admissions. We took a much more proactive attitude, hunting through charts, even checking on kids while they slept. This was much different from waiting for pagers to blare, which was what residents did at every other hospital I knew.

I was clueless on call at Children's. One night, a little boy with a urethral disorder was screaming in agony.

"I can't peeeee!! I can't peeeeeeeeeeeeeeeeee!!!" he wailed. He obviously needed a urethral catheter in order to relieve the pressure in his bladder. I panicked. I had never inserted a urethral catheter, even in an adult. I wasn't about to place one in a child with rearranged anatomy after multiple surgeries for urinary problems. I called for help from my senior resident who did the job for me.

I didn't know how to evaluate the next patient. He had had a blackout, and could not give an accurate history of events. He was obviously anxious, but seemed physically unharmed per my examination, so I ordered his hard cervical collar to be removed. The following morning, the attending, who was the chief of the division (that is, the most highly regarded doc in the hospital), dressed me down in front of my peers:

"You mean to tell me that no one did a rectal exam?" she said, glaring at me. "This boy couldn't give you a history, and you didn't do a *rectal* exam?" I would have given anything just to disappear.

I didn't know how to consult a specialist.

I didn't know how to use the hospital phones.

I didn't know anything.

When lunchtime rolled around, I rarely ate because I was usually in a pimp session (being questioned about medical trivia in a group setting by an attending) or talking to a parent or finally bumping into a specialist I had been missing all week. The Children's residents all knew each other, the nurses, the attendings and the system. They could instantly calculate pediatric dosing for any medication. When I needed to get something done, I would smile and nervously ask a nurse to help me, and then be met with raised eyebrows and a vague half-answer. Sometimes, there was a helpful resident or nurse. But often, as I searched for the right person or correct procedure that would have been apparent to anyone around me, I was completely ignored and left to battle the unfamiliar hospital alone.

The biggest blessing/curse of all: the Big-City Med Students (BCMS). They had perfectly pressed short white coats and young beautiful faces with sparkling smiles and attitudes, still guided by the search for approval by authority figures. When I "taught" these BCMS at Children's, I allowed (yes, *allowed,* since they *begged* to do my work for me, to have responsibilities, anything to demonstrate their intelligence to get a medical brownie point) them to write my notes for me, take the patient histories and even put orders in for me. It was embarrassing. Each day at Children's, we walked through the halls en masse (attending, several residents, a pharmacist, a group of BCMS and nurses), saw patient after patient and determined the treatment plan for each child. Each new attending of the week pimped us individually, and the BCMS who pranced along with us cheerfully chirped the perfect answers to the questions, while I just stood there, feeling dumber than a dirt clod. If I had had a tail, it would have been between my legs. It was painfully obvious that they had had superior training, and that I did not belong.

Day after day, I lived in perpetual fear of losing my residency spot. I imagined it hundreds of times. The cluster of us white coats would be walking down the pristine halls, doing our rounds of the sick kids, and my pager would suddenly emit a piercing tone. The music in the saloon would stop. Everyone would look up from their clipboards and laptops to stare at me. I would stumble off to the nearest phone, and punch in the numbers. When Dr. Hampton (my program director) answered, he would explain that he had received complaints about me from Children's attendings, residents and even the pediatric nurses. They all could see I was not prepared for an inpatient pediatric rotation, let alone a career in medicine. He would ask for me to be removed from the rotation immediately, and to remediate. What was to be remediated changed depending on the intensity of my insecurity — sometimes I was to repeat the rotation, sometimes intern year, sometimes the previous four years of medical school.

Every day I answered questions in the vaguest possible way, trying to fake my way through, until I could scramble and read about the topics at home. I was struck by the fact that I was actually a "doctor" at this point — I was Dr. Southwick, the dumbest doctor in the world. I watched the attending's face tense up when it was my turn to talk, bracing herself for my idiotic case presentation.

I began to lose weight. I gradually stopped enjoying even my tiny amount of time off each week. Time off became just more empty space to think about how stupid I was, and what a terrible doctor I was becoming.

Then the nausea started. I took more frequent trips to the bathroom just to catch my breath, splash water on my face and try to get my bearings.

I was in a constant state of anxiety and dread. My heart would be pounding when I went to bed, and pounding when I woke up. In the morning, I would wake up in a pitch-black cold apartment, then my alarm would go off like a gun starting the race of my day. I would go through my morning routine. Whether I ate breakfast or not, I would gag, and eventually vomit. I would kiss Jude goodbye and tell myself to muscle through it, that it wouldn't last forever. I could do this.

At one point, I confided my distress to my friend Edith (from the beach vacation), who was an neurosurgical resident. She laughed.

"Oh yeah! In the mornings, right?" she shouted, and pretended as if she were gagging. That made me feel better. It was comforting that at least I wasn't the only one.

I drove to the hospital every morning, planning to get a computer to myself and review all the patient details before the others, to try to get a head start and have at least one piece of information to contribute to the team rounding. But no matter how early I arrived, the med students would be there already, bright-eyed and ready to spout off the vital signs, top 10 differential diagnosis list and favorite color of every patient.

Then came the crying. I would come home after work and make myself flashcards of all the material I needed to learn (from little notes over the course of the day). I would fall asleep around 11 PM, and when the alarm went off at 3:30 or 4:00 AM

I would burst into tears. I hyperventilated, sobbed and gagged until I vomited, then pack up my backpack and march out to my car in the dark, storming into another day, feeling utterly useless.

After what seemed like a hundred mornings of this sad routine, Jude stopped putting on a happy face and simply asked what she could do. She was starting to feel my desperation.

"Should I drive you to work?" she asked.

So she started driving me to work. That didn't help.

"Should I plan out your day for you?"

She wrote out my day, minute by minute, so I would have a little day map in my pocket. It seemed to make things worse.

"Should I get your mom?" she asked.

At this point I was on the bathroom floor in fetal position. I couldn't breathe or eat or talk. I sobbed, and I nodded.

My mom arrived for a weeklong stay, and it was a solemn, somber visit — as if she had come for my funeral. She cooked for us, and tried to be supportive in any possible way. It was the sweetest gesture, and I was so grateful to her, but it didn't help my situation. I still hyperventilated, vomited and sobbed before work. I still felt I was worthless, marking time until I was booted out of the program and would have to look for another career. Every day Jude and my mom drove me to and from work, trying to remove any possible shred of extra stress I had. It was so kind of them, but it didn't help.

Nothing helped.

Eventually, the rotation ended.

I later discovered that the entire Children's residency, as well as the BCMS, had been given an Intern Survival Guide specifically for inpatient pediatrics floors. It contained all the information I had needed: the consult names and numbers, vital signs for different ages, how to calculate a drip rate, treatment plans for different disease processes — all the answers to all of my questions. Everyone had received a guide at the beginning of the rotation.

Everyone...except me, and the other family medicine residents.

A few weeks later, I met with our family medicine program's pediatric adviser and asked about the survival guide. I received my copy seven months after the rotation ended. On a positive note, family medicine interns now receive them before starting the rotation.

The next day, my rotation at Magee Womens Hospital started.

HOW TIRING IS RESIDENCY?

So tiring.

When Jude and I went out to eat, I avoided ordering salad; I didn't have the energy to chew that much.

I passed out twice over the three years (once while walking out of a patient room at Shadyside after a discussion with a patient about her blood transfusion, once at Magee while examining newborns in the nursery) as a result of fatigue, caffeine overuse, dehydration and stress.

Many days in residency impaired me more than when I was drunk. The amount of output was so immense, it was hard to catch up. I would fall asleep while dictating. I always stuttered at the same locations in a dictation, I suppose because that's around the time my brain was trying to shut down to sleep.

I had always functioned best with nine to 10 hours of sleep, so those long days and nights in the hospital really took their toll on me. In medical school, one of my childhood friends came for a visit and Jude asked him what I was like when I was a kid.

"Frances was really...um...*sleepy*," he said.

If I sat down for just a few seconds at home, I would immediately fall asleep — because I was so exhausted. It became common that when I didn't sleep in a 24-hour-shift, I would come home wired for a couple of hours, so Jude and I used this as catch-up and breakfast time. The problem was that I desperately needed rest as well as proper nutrition. I was so lacking in both these areas that I developed a tremor. I had lost weight and had muscle pain, so when I would lie down my whole body would ache. But it would only last for a few seconds... before I was asleep again.

Not only the fatigue but the uncertainty of working in so many different environments made me insecure. I questioned myself frequently and worked hard to keep up. Interestingly, the very small things became more important to me, and to my fellow residents. One particular anecdote sums up the experience quite well. I knew a resident whose partner packed her lunch each day; usually a sandwich, an apple, a box of crackers and some type of dessert. One day, unbeknownst to my resident friend, they had run out of apples. She happened to have worked 130 hours that week and came home crying on the last day. She said the thing that would have helped her was that apple; her final day was shattered because that single comfort was missing; she looked forward to it like a friend.

All these factors contribute to an unhealthy state of mind. I was depressed, which further compounded my fatigue. A common sign of depression is sleeping frequently; it's not a conscious decision, but a symptom of mental/physical collapse. Poor Jude. If she began telling me a story about her day, I would fall asleep. Her voice relaxed me. My brain would sift through the information and ask, "Is this data vital for a patient situation or pimp session? No? Then OK, I'm out."

Some days, I could handle all of it and stay energized. Most of the time, though, this was not the case. I would sit at my laptop to type patient notes and end up staring at the screen, then typing a bit, and then staring again. I believe I was coming in and out of Stage 1 sleep. I would refocus every few moments, but I'm not sure how long those lapses lasted; probably between a few seconds and a few minutes.

My problem was not unique, of course. Working long hours without sleep has always been a problem in medical training. The issue was finally addressed in 2003 (before I was a resident), when the rules for resident work hours changed from unlimited to 80 hours a week. However, there is still much debate about how much weight these rules hold. Most studies of whether the 80-hour-work-week show that it has not improved things that much, namely, patient safety.

Perhaps it's because residents work longer than 80 hours anyway.

Perhaps it's because of all the other constraints they must conform to outside the 80 hours.

Or perhaps it's because 80 hours is **still too many hours**, especially in such an intense environment.

Many of the older instructors who trained under the unlimited work-hour schedule maintain the mindset of how they were trained, just like folks who have been through military training. It's the "If I went through it, you should too" mentality, and it's just human nature. Today, residents are required to report their work hours and all residency programs must follow the work-hour rules or risk being shut down. And that's the dilemma. If a program closes, its residents are forced to uproot midway and move to another city, if there is a residency slot open for him/her them all. So the hours that residents work can still be a bit murky. That is why I lied on my work hours to make them fit nicely into the boxes; I wanted to stay at Shadyside. I liked the faculty and fellow residents, and I didn't want to start over in another hospital system. The "mistakes" I made early on in reporting my work hours were "caught in time" by the administrative staff, and I was asked to sign off on the "corrections." I know that my friend Edith personally logged 136 hours one week, but reported her maximum of "80." You do what is necessary to keep going.

After my intern year, one of the administrators held a meeting, notifying residents of a new set of rules in the works (now in effect) to improve conditions for interns. Interns would be limited to maximum 16-consecutive-hour shifts (instead of 30-hour shifts). The 80 hour rule would still be in effect. There would be no change in the rules for second- or third-year residents.

"Well, I don't see how it is going to improve things. We know from the studies, medical errors did not improve after the current work-hour restrictions were imposed," he said matter-of-factly.

We all looked at one another. The news was not surprising — everyone lies about their hours.

"The only metric that improved was deaths of residents and others involved in resident-caused motor vehicle accidents. So we are not hopeful that these work-hour rules will be meaningful," the administrator said, without emotion. I guess that metric wasn't significant to him.

Friends and acquaintances outside the medical community regarded my training (and my mental/physical state) with a mixture of emotions. I often asked people to repeat their sentences and had long, halting response times in conversation. I would explain that I was fatigued because I worked long hours and seldom slept, so I needed more time to process things. Sometimes I gave details about my workload, to help them understand. People were confused.

They would respond with disbelief:

"I can't believe that — are you making this up?"

Or anger:

"Why does it have to be like this? What is wrong with the world? That fucking hospital!"

Or pity:

"You poor thing."

Or shame:

"I feel sick that we are such terrible people, making our young doctors go through this hell."

Or fear:

"God, I wonder what my doctor went through…"

CONSEQUENCES OF CHRONIC SLEEP LOSS

Sleep deprivation, which has been well studied, impairs human functioning on many levels.

This is what we know:

1. Lack of sleep affects motor skills, cognitive performance and mood. Of these three metrics, mood is the most significantly affected. (Pilcher, Vol 19(4), May 1996)

2. Related to overall functioning, partial sleep deprivation (frequently interrupted sleep) is more damaging than long-term or short-term sleep deprivation. (Pilcher, Vol 19(4), May 1996)

3. Sleep-deprived people are more aggressive toward their partners. (Keller, Vol 23(4), 2014)

4. Chronic sleep loss can lead to depression. (Vandale, Vol 166(2))

5. Sleep is essential for memory consolidation and decision making. (Vandale, Vol 166(2))

6. Sleep-deprived individuals speak less clearly and have longer temporal order judgment thresholds (takes them longer to remember which object came first, after being

presented with two objects in succession). (Fostick, June 2014, Vol 57(3))

7. After a long shift, medical interns are 2.5 times more likely to have motor vehicle accidents. (Blosser, 2005)

8. Partially sleep-deprived people cannot reliably gauge how sleepy or impaired they are. That is, even as they get less sleep and their mental functioning performance scores drop, they don't know they are getting sleepier. They don't notice their cognitive abilities deteriorating. (College, 2010)

PREPPING FOR MAGEE WOMENS HOSPITAL

I assumed I would be expected to deliver babies, but I wasn't completely clear on the details.

The weekend before I started working at Magee Womens Hospital, I pulled out the OB for Family Medicine book I received in Orientation Week. I only had 24 hours to read, so I wanted pointers on specific topics to review.

I called Orlando, one of my trusted senior residents.

"So, what should I study before I start at Magee?"

"Everything," he said. "You know, everything related to delivery. The mechanics of delivery, the emergency meds, examining a newborn. Once they see that you know what you're doing, they'll let you in on more deliveries. That's what happened to me. I jumped on this one delivery and the attending let me follow him all day! I picked up three more! Don't worry. Just think back to your deliveries in med school."

I thought back. I had "delivered" a whopping *two* babies.

My first experience was quite memorable. It was Thanksgiving and I was working in the ED. My attending was a goofy, stereotypical ER doctor: He was loud and funny, and thrived on fast pace. I was trying to make sure I wasn't in the way, and to help as much as I could. I was told to see a new patient in Room 3. With pen and paper in hand, decked out in my short white coat clanging with instruments, I approached the patient, a 20-something woman, who looked uncomfortable. The triage note said, "ABDOMINAL PAIN."

She had normal vital signs.

"Hi, I'm student Dr. Southwick," I said. "What brings you in this evening?"

"My stomach hurts. I think I have some really bad gas."

"Okay, when did this start?"

"Tonight."

"Anything else?"

"No, my stomach just really hurts. I think I am going to be sick."

I examined her, and went out to present her case to the goofy attending.

"When was her last period?" he asked.

"Last month."

"Does she have any vaginal discharge?"

"Um, I...didn't ask."

"Jesus. You didn't ask? She's a 24-year-old female with belly pain and you don't know?"

He examined her, then came back to get me.

"She has discharge," he said. "Ready for the gyne exam?"

The nurses moved her to the gyne room. My attending and I walked in, and he rolled up on his stool to examine her vagina. Within a few seconds, his face went white, then bright red. He swung around to scream at me, *"CALL THE LABOR SUITE!!! CALL THEM!!!"*

I panicked a little. Labor suite? Of course, I didn't know the number. I didn't even know where it was in the hospital.

That rotation wasn't for another three months! One of the nurses called the number and handed me the receiver. What was I supposed to say? Just then the attending yelled:

"I SEE A HEAD!!! GET HER UP THERE!!!"

"Hello? Oh, yes, hello...um...this is...um...student Dr. Southwick in the Emergency Room. Um..."

"TELL THEM IT'S A BABY, AND IT'S COMING NOW! DO THEY WANT HER HERE, OR UP THERE?"

"We have a baby...uh... a woman who is in labor right now, do you..."

"SEND HER UP!" everyone shouted.

My attending decided it would be a better learning experience for me to go up and assist with the delivery rather than hang around the ED looking for work, so I accompanied her with the transport team. On the elevator up to the Labor Suite, I asked the patient her estimated date of delivery, her OB history, and when her last ultrasound was. She looked bewildered, claiming she didn't know she was pregnant, and that she had been getting her period every month.

When we got to the Labor Suite, the charge nurse asked me, "How far along is she?"

"She doesn't...I mean...I don't know," I said.

"What do you mean? How many weeks? What are her G's and P's?"

Oh boy. This was going to be a long night.

The nurse smacked on a latex glove and lubed it up, then proceeded to examine the patient.

"She's 6," she stated, referring to centimeters of cervical dilation. "Get the ultrasound."

The ultrasound showed that the baby was breech (meaning it was butt first, rather than head first; this can be a dangerous situation, especially if the team is unprepared). The nurses really got on the horn, then. They decided to prep for an emergency C-section. The OB doc on call still wasn't there. I half-realized that I was the one with a white coat on.

"Go get gowned up!" the nurse barked. "The doctor will be here any minute!"

I went off in search of gowning-up garb. I hadn't had my surgical rotation yet. I had a faint memory from a lecture the year before about what I would need. After a few minutes, I found the locker room and the necessary attire in little boxes scattered throughout the room. I covered my shoes with blue shoe covers, my hair with a blue cap, my body with a white "bunny suit" (usually reserved for baby daddies, or internists who don't own scrubs anymore but are coming to observe a surgery for a day, or psychiatrists who otherwise would never set foot in an OR except to perform electroconvulsive therapy). I remembered to grab a blue mask, too. I fumbled around outside the OR in my outfit, trying to figure out how to "scrub in" when the attending arrived, breathless, limping.

"Doesn't sound like there's time for that. You ready? Let's go!"

He slapped on a scrub cap, pulled on some knee-length boot-like shoe covers and a mask, quickly soaped and rinsed instead of performing the formal scrubbing-in ritual, and stormed into the room. I followed.

During the delivery, my jobs were to:

1. Retract (hold the skin back with a large metal instrument, in order to show the surgeon the organs), and

2. Hold my hand under the doctor's face to catch sweat drops so they wouldn't fall into the sterile field. (This was a very unusual emergency surgery, and would not have normally been part of my duties, but the air conditioner wasn't working well, the doctor was very large and we had a serious situation at hand. This lead to his profuse sweating.)

Over the next five minutes, I saw: the baby being pulled out violently; the mother's inverted uterus; and the baby's wet-behind-the-ears dad crying, completely stupified, in the hallway. I also learned that in a delivery I should always wear knee-high boot covers like the doctor. After that, I nearly passed out from the heat and anxiety.

My other "delivery" was a vaginal birth that occurred on my actual OB/GYN rotation my third year of medical school. I was instructed to "labor with her." Translation: I uneasily walked into the patient room, talked to the mother-to-be and her family for a few minutes, looked through her chart, stared at her strip (contraction pattern coupled with baby's heart rate), and planned what to do in case the attending didn't arrive. Then I walked out and sat with the nurses for 30 minutes, and read about obstetrics. I went back and forth like this about 20 times, for hours. When delivery seemed imminent, the nurse paged the attending. He presented himself, all smiles, and we delivered the baby with the help of a Kiwi vacuum (a suction cup attached to the baby's head).

Back to residency land.

I continued my conversation with Orlando, asking for more tips.

"Okay, Orlando, are there any top pointers you would recommend?"

"Just get your numbers," he said. "Make sure you get at least past 25 and you should be golden until second year."

I quickly learned that quantity ("my numbers"), not quality, was the way to complete this rotation successfully. I had eight total weeks (four in intern year and four in second year) to get my numbers (that is, deliver 40 babies). What counted as a "delivery" was in flux depending upon the attending of the day. Some said I had to actually deliver the baby, which seemed reasonable at first. But as the days passed, I started to appreciate the more pragmatic attendings' opinions that as long as I was present, it was counted as a delivery.

MAGEE

I woke up to my alarm at 3:30 AM on Monday, the first day of my Magee Womens Hospital rotation. As I drove there, I was shaking and my nausea was starting.

What am I doing? I know almost nothing about delivering babies. Yes, I had four weeks of OB/GYN over a year ago, but what did I actually learn? To measure a pregnant belly, and count the number of fetal heart tones in a minute?

I mentally went through the seven "cardinal" movements a baby goes through in the delivery process.

Engagement, descent, flexion...then what? External rotation? Extension?

I was wired; my hands tightly gripped the steering wheel. I was almost there.

Where do I park?

I hadn't planned this out very well.

I circled the hospital a few times, and found a place where I could swipe my resident badge. Voila! The gate to the parking lot opened. I parked my car and walked toward the hospital. Once inside, I had no idea where I was going. In Orientation Week, hadn't they told us where the family medicine office was?

After 20 minutes of wandering down hallways and stairwells and asking five nurses and administrative assistants, I finally found the family medicine office. I had heard that the Magee family medicine office was once a call room, and that the family medicine call room had been a closet. This explained both why I couldn't find the office and the opinion that the physicians and nurses at Magee held of family medicine.

I spotted Brad, my senior resident for the day. He was from St. Margaret's, and I was instantly grateful that I knew him. We had worked together in my fourth year of med school. He was a laid-back, snowboarder/surfer type, wearing a sweatshirt over his scrubs. His face was unshaven, his hair was wet from his shower, and he was wearing glasses, a backup for his usual contact lenses.

"Frances! You're starting this morning? Great! Good for you, you found the place. That's half the battle on the first day," he said with a hearty smile.

I laughed nervously. I was absolutely terrified. It was 5:50 AM and pitch black.

Sign-in consisted of the overnight resident pointing at the "Board." The Board displayed a list of patient names and details. It was large and white, covering most of a wall, scored with black electrical tape. The overnight resident spoke in medical lingo to Brad, the senior resident coming on for the day.

"Okay, so you got five in. First one's an AB positive with antibodies prime who PROM'd and went for a stat section. Her baby's a Klammerhigh. 9 and 9, haven't done the red reflex yet. She wants him circ'd. Next one is a multip with no FOB. She was GBS positive, pen allergic, so she got vanc. She smoked the whole pregnancy. She's been having some lates, so we got MFM. Number three is a 40-year-old G4P2 with no prenatal care. She's measuring 37 and she's a TOLAC hoping for VBAC. Do you know how to put in an IUPC?"

Oh, God.

The next 12 hours were a blur. Brad whizzed me around the hospital and talked so much with such a bulk of new information, I thought I would explode. *New attending every day. Sign up for deliveries, but not on the patients in red; those belong to OB residents. DO NOT sign up for a patient until rounds are over. Once your lady gets to 8, stay in the room. Send your notes to the attending before first rounds. There are safety rounds (announcements of all the patients in labor and their details) every four hours. Follow at least two patients laboring at a time. Ask families if you can be their resident, call the attending and follow the chart. Get a pickle phone* (we used hospital-bound cordless phones instead of pagers at Magee) *and put your number on your patient's white board. Get your scrubs from the scrub-dispensing machine using a code* (completely new concept to me at this point), *and make sure you return them on the opposite side of the machine when you leave. Remember that the stairwell you need is the one at the end of the hall. Do NOT speak unless spoken to in safety rounds. One of the residents carries the triage phone at all times, and responds to it no matter WHAT is happening. See your babies and moms before the first rounds start. Massage the hell out of the uterus. Teach the moms to use an alcohol wipe around the umbilical cord every day[3]. Remember that bloody vaginal discharge from a newborn female is normal. Use your thumb to open the newborn's eye. And above all, get your numbers.*

By the end of the day, I was overwhelmed and confused, but was proud of myself — I scored one delivery. I had stood near the foot of the bed through a vaginal delivery of one of my

---

3 Now an obsolete practice.

fellow residents' patients. My attending that day was easy on us, so he counted it as a delivery for all present.

I drove home, stuck my key in the lock, and walked inside. Jude was in the living room, reading. She looked up from her book and searched my eyes expectantly.

"How was it, Honey? How was your first day delivering babies?"

"I don't know. It was good. I love you."

We ate dinner. I reviewed as much OB info as I could, and fell asleep around 11.

Up at 3:30 AM.

The next day I got home at 10:30 PM. Earlier in the evening I had jumped onto a case of a family medicine patient. The attending was Dr. Anderson, an exuberant woman with an enormous passion for obstetrics. I had seen Dr. Anderson get her feelings hurt by residents who didn't share her enthusiasm. Those hurt feelings naturally resulted in Dr. Anderson talking negatively about these residents to other faculty and residents. I didn't want to be on her bad resident list. That night she was excitedly teaching me details of laboring, and explained that she never left a woman while she was in labor. She walked a pregnant teenager around the room, bounced on a yoga ball with her, and breathed with her. Dr. Anderson taught me how to check a cervix and write a good OB patient note. She had given me so much of her time that I felt both excited to be learning so much and obligated to stay until the baby was dry and the delivery paperwork was completed. Went to bed at midnight.

Next day: up at 3:30 again.

By the end of the week, I had lost another inch or so in the waist.

I attempted to sign up for patients but was edged out of deliveries by BCMS, was looked upon with disdain and disgust by OB nurses, OB attendings, OB residents and staff members. I didn't know why yet, but it slowly became clear that most people here hated family medicine people, and specifically hated family medicine residents most of all.

That weekend I was on call, on my own. There was no family medicine attending in the hospital. No senior resident. A friendly family medicine attending had assured me, "We are not immediately available on weekends, but we have an agreement with the OB docs. They will help you and supervise you, and if your patient goes into labor, we will come in. Page the on-call family medicine attending once you have a plan with the OB attending."

My triage phone rang. It was a nurse calling me to the triage area for a new family medicine case. She had vaginal discharge and pain. I evaluated the patient as best I could. Then I walked out to the nurse's station, and had to beg an OB attending to teach me how to evaluate her.

"Don't your attendings teach you anything?" he asked with a snarl. He stormed into the patient room, elbowing me out of the way, and performed the sterile examination.

"Where is your attending, anyway? Why are you asking me?"

I didn't know what to say. My face turned red, and my heart pumped hard and fast straight to my stomach.

I thought there was an agreement? Was he not aware? Was I asking the wrong attending?

Up at 4 AM the next day, back to Magee by 5:30 to park, up to the family medicine office by 5:50 to review labs and new patients. I rounded, came back to safety rounds, saw triage patients, signed up for patients, stood around waiting, paged attendings who ignored me, was kicked out of rooms by midwives and families. I was a spider circling the drain. I walked down to the bathroom and sat on the toilet, my legs sticking to the seat. I held my head in my hands and grimaced, squeezing tears out of my eyes.

The next day was the same story. More of the same — feeling in the way, out of my element, clueless.

I slept on call with the triage phone hanging on the doorknob of the call room because the reception was better there. It rang, waking me abruptly from restless sleep. I jumped off the bed and grabbed the phone.

"Family medicine?" the voice asked.

"Yes."

"You've got an IU [muffled words] in 3."

"Excuse me?" I said.

The reception was so poor that I could barely hear the voice, so I went out into the hallway.

"You have a patient in Room 3," the annoyed caller repeated. Then the line went dead.

I stuck the phone in the scrub pocket of my shirt and walked down to the triage area. I pulled the paper chart out and surveyed the scribbled information supplied by the nurse on duty. The patient was a 19-year-old female, and this was her first pregnancy. She was full term, 40 weeks along, and in labor. Easy enough. In the exam room, I found the patient on the OB gurney, looking calm and relaxed.

"Hi, I'm Dr. Southwick, one of the family medicine doctors. How are you tonight?"

The woman, a thin African-American teen, smiled and rubbed her belly.

"I'm good, Doc," she said. "The contractions are starting to hurt, though."

I looked at her monitors. The contractions had a normal pattern, early labor. The monitor for the baby's heart was off.

"Let me adjust this for you," I said, replacing the fetal heart monitor. I strapped it in place and checked the wires, but there was nothing on the screen. I grabbed the ultrasound lubricant to get a better reading. Again, nothing.

I spent a few minutes getting more medical history, then went to the nurse's station and asked the patient's nurse to help me with the fetal heart monitor. She stared at me, arms crossed.

"I told you. It's an IUFD."

"Okay, what does that mean?"

"Intrauterine fetal demise," she said with a scoff.

The baby was dead, but no one had told the patient yet.

I waited a few minutes, trying to figure out what to do. I decided to page the on-call family medicine attending.

"Yes?"

"Hi Dr. Wenz, it's Frances. I have an IUFD and I'm not sure what to do."

"OK, well, talk her through it and I'll be there in a few hours."

I tried to get more specific information.

"Listen, I'll be there in a few hours," he said. "Just put in the orders the OB residents use."

I walked back to the patient's room.

"When was the last time you felt your baby move?" I asked.

She thought for a few seconds, and said,

"About an hour or two."

I told her that I had some bad news and asked if she would like to have a relative or friend present in the room.

"Why? What's wrong?" she said.

"I need to talk to you about your baby."

She called her mother in. I told them that the baby's heart had stopped, and that there was nothing we could do.

They became tearful, then furious.

"What? She was fine this afternoon! We were just at the doctor's today!"

"I know this is difficult news to take," I said. "I will be here with you through this."

I went into the hallway, stunned. I could hear the patient and her mother weeping behind the door.

I worked through the night and into the next day, trying to help her accept that her baby was dead, and that no one knew why. The daytime attending and I delivered the baby vaginally. For an hour after the delivery, the patient cried as she held and rocked her dead infant.

I went to the bathroom. I was so exhausted, I couldn't think. I was drowning in this hospital. I punched one thigh, and then the other one. I punched them as hard as I could. It made me feel somewhat better. It was a little release.

By the end of the second week, I had lost so much weight and had been on my feet so long that it really hurt to lay down in bed. Everything hurt. I was back to throwing up and crying in the mornings. I was running on half my usual sleep and food intake. But I kept showing up.

That second weekend, I was on call on Sunday. Daytime call. That meant my attending would be there for a few morning hours until we finished rounding, and I would stay until the night resident came on. I arrived at the usual time, unlocked the door and looked up at the Board. It was full. Eight postpartums with babies, and two in labor. This meant 16 patients to round on and two to labor with. Plus, I had the triage pager and was the only family medicine resident in the hospital. This was going to be impossible.

Dr. Anderson didn't get in until 11 AM; she was rounding at Shadyside Hospital first. I had paged her, asking a few pressing questions. Finally she came, after I had rounded on half of the patients. I missed safety rounds.

Dr. Anderson has quirks. One of them is that cannot stop teaching. She talked and talked while I kept trying to round and finish patient notes. She wanted to teach me how to approach fever in the newborn, how to help with post-partum depression, how to insert an IUPC (device to monitor contractions internally).

The triage phone rang, and at the same time I got a page about a patient in labor. I excused myself from the room to answer the calls. An OB attending in the hall gave me a weird look.

"Why weren't you at safety rounds? You have two in labor."

Dr. Anderson overheard and came out of the room.

"You have somebody in triage too? OK, Frances, we just have to put out fires. You're scared because you have no senior right? I'll be your senior. Don't worry! Go! You have to go see the patient! Get in there!"

I ran down to the triage room where a teenager in labor was bleeding. I paged Dr. Anderson again.

The day went on like this. No matter where I was, I was supposed to be somewhere else. Dr. Anderson ended up discharging two patients for me. I felt like an epic failure.

"I don't know what's wrong with me! I am trying, I'm just so behind. I'm sorry. Thank you for helping me," I told her.

"Don't worry, Frances," she said. "You're just sooooo slow! Do you think you could speed it up a little? I'm here for you! But we gotta do this!"

I could see how disappointed she was. I went to take care of one of the laboring patients, and the nurse physically edged me out as I was instructing the patient on labor breathing.

"Pay attention to *ME*," she instructed the patient, "*I* am your birth coach." She glared at me, irritated that I was interfering with *her* patient. I left the room.

I couldn't keep this up. I went to the bathroom and beat the shit out of my thighs. I wished I could escape. Escape. Why hadn't I gone into sign language? I could have been an interpreter. There was no way to leave. I wished I could just jump off a building.

I went back to the family medicine office and stopped short of the door. I heard Dr. Anderson on the phone talking about me to her husband. She said that I wasn't keeping up, that she would be home very late. Could he please bring the kids by the hospital so she could hug them goodnight?

I am a dead weight around her ankles.

I sat in the stairwell for a few minutes to compose myself and allow her to complete the phone call. I walked back to the family medicine office.

"Anyone laboring?" Dr. Anderson said.

"No, not right now," I replied.

She hunched down in her chair and faced me full-on. She stared into my eyes.

"What is going on with you?"

She was so intense. I couldn't keep it in.

"I don't know what's wrong with me! I can't keep up! There is too much! I am too stupid to be in this program. I can't handle it!"

She nodded, and kept staring.

"Are you feeling depressed?" she asked.

"I have lost so much weight. Everything hurts. The days here are bad and I can't sleep, but the weekends and the hours off are worse. I just keep going over everything in my mind, how stupid I am. How many things I have probably missed. Everyone hates me here. I couldn't handle Children's and I know I can't handle this. I can't focus. I can't even read anymore."

She kept her serious tone.

"Have you thought about taking an antidepressant?"

This idea had occurred to me, but my family's judgment of people on antidepressants deterred me. Plus, Jude's family was obsessed with taking pills for various illnesses including habit-forming "happy pills." She was 100 percent against taking medicine for mood disorders. Plus, my problem seemed to be my own inadequacy, not a chemical imbalance.

"I don't want to do that," I said.

Dr. Anderson recounted her bout of crippling depression during medical school, and how a friend of hers "literally carried her to a psychiatrist's office" who prescribed an antidepressant.

"It saved my life," she said. "I call it vitamin C. C for Celexa."

The next day, I felt like I could hardly breathe. I couldn't eat. I couldn't sleep.

I called her for the prescription.

MAGEE, THE THIRD WEEKEND

Golden weekends (a whole weekend off — from Friday at sign-out through Monday at sign-in) were worse for me — more time for feelings to bubble up. The third weekend of Magee Womens Hospital was my first golden weekend in two months. Jude was out of town, recording a CD.

As a distraction from myself, I called John.

I had seen him two nights earlier, when we had had a late dinner at a Thai restaurant. That is, he ate and I tried to eat, as tears flowed down my face and I shook with anxiety and nausea.

"I'm thinking about jumping off buildings," I told him. "I can't get it out of my head. I look up methods of suicide between patients."

He stopped chewing and looked up from his pad Thai.

"Really?" he said, with concern.

Beat of silence.

"Frances, do you...do you want...an intervention here?"

I shrugged, not knowing what to say. I asked for a to-go bag, packed up my dinner and hugged him goodnight.

So when I called him now, two days later, he wanted to see me again because he was worried about me. We spent a couple of hours together walking around a strip mall, then circled the nearby movie theater a few times. We talked and reminisced about the eight years we had known each other.

After leaving John, I know I drove home because I ended up back at our apartment, but I don't remember the drive. I could hardly walk through the door because my legs felt as heavy as cement. I dragged myself to bed. I had such little energy, it was even a chore to cry. I don't remember much about the night, but there was no sleep. All I could think about was ending my life.

Jump. Jump. Jump. Jump. Jump. Jump.

As the sun rose on Sunday, I was still shuddering. My vision was partly obscured by tears and mucus. I knew I had to jump today — before Jude got home.

I wanted to hear someone's voice before I died.

At 8:00, I called John. No answer.

I dialed Dr. Anderson's number. She answered in a groggy voice. I couldn't keep my cool. I confided that I was not doing well and asked if she thought the Celexa she had prescribed was making my suicidal thoughts worse; I had been taking it for almost a week. She dismissed this as a non-possibility, explaining that she thought the medicine hadn't started working yet. She asked me to call back at noon, and I agreed. She instructed me to go outside and take a walk.

After I hung up, I realized there were still a few hours to make my plan work. On a scratch piece of paper, I wrote out a last note to Jude and my parents. It read:

Hi everyone!

There was nothing more that could have been done! That's all there is to it. ☺ I am so, ~~soo~~ so sorry for your loss but I was dragging everyone down and not enjoying life. It's no way to live, the way I've been feeling for so long — even before residency. I only blame myself — there is nothing you could have done, I can assure you. Please ~~tko~~ take to heart the 4 Agreements and don't take it personally. This was about me, not you. I love you all but there is nothing more to do, but say goodbye. Thank you for the love and support. If I were reading this, I would want so much more from Shadyside Honda this letter! ☺

I love you. ♡
& Frances

5'21 [REDACTED] Ave

I grabbed Jude's favorite sweatshirt, a second-hand green-and-gray Abercrombie & Fitch, out of the dirty laundry and pulled it over my head. I grabbed the car keys and started driving in search of the highest bridge I could find, perhaps the same bridge Ronald Fletcher had mentioned when dealing with a suicidal patient.

Ronald was the family medicine department's wise therapist/social worker, who gave the residents lectures on psychosocial health topics. I overheard him telling Dr. Carter, our department's kind faculty psychiatrist, about a patient who had stopped on the 40th Street Bridge and dangled her legs over the edge, contemplating her jump. To dissuade her from a future suicide attempt, Ronald said that he had described to the patient what the water would feel like: how it would be freezing and would choke the life out of her, unceremoniously. He explained to her that her family would be forced to identify her battered, bloated, unrecognizable body after it had been fished out of the river. (I imagined Jude's reaction but thought she would at least be comforted to find me in the A&F sweatshirt.) He commented on how shocked and concerned he was about the patient's actions. I was surprised by his strong emotional response — didn't he hear this shit every day? And now, my thoughts were almost identical to hers...

In the car, I called Jude. She sounded happy. She talked about some flowers she was noticing — or maybe that was me talking about some flowers I remembered. I drove toward the Allegheny River. I got lost and didn't care. I wished Jude well on her day — somehow I was able to be calmer with her than with Dr. Anderson. Jude didn't pick up on anything different in my voice — maybe she was used to it because I had been depressed for several weeks.

I considered a few bridges. Any of them would be easy enough to park near, walk to and jump from. I settled on the 40th Street Bridge. If Ronald was concerned about his patient jumping, it must be high enough.

I parked at the precipice and sat for a second. I opened the door and felt the cool air. I walked onto the bridge and looked down at the dark, swirling water.

My cellphone rang.

Dr. Anderson.

It was 10:16 — too early to talk to her — why was she jumping the gun?

I flicked the phone open.

"Hello."

"Hi Frances, it's Dr. Anderson. Just thought I would see how your day was going."

"Okay."

"Where are you?"

Did she hear the cars passing?

"The north side." I lied. I had no idea was part of town this was called.

"Is that where you decided to take a walk?" she asked.

No answer on my part.

"You're not scoping out bridges are you?" Her mention of bridges pierced my chest.

Again, I didn't answer her. I was stunned. My brain clumsily scanned for memory fragments. Had I mentioned bridges to her?

"Why don't you come back to my neighborhood?" she said. "I was planning on going for a walk anyway. You know the entrance to Frick Park..."

I let her ramble on. My head was swimming. I was exhausted and confused, and I didn't plan to meet her anyhow.

"I think I'm just going to go home," I said.

She asked me several more times to join her and I declined again.

"I'm lost and I need to find my way home."

I was pissed now. Why had I even called her? Why had I ever agreed to be a resident?

Several minutes of silence.

"Frances, it's not going to make it easier for anyone if you end your life."

I sank inside myself. I knew I had get myself back to our apartment. I knew I had to distract myself there until my next shift knocked me back into panicky work mode rather than hysterical suicidal mode.

The next week:

1. I bought Dr. Anderson a giant chocolate bar (to keep her quiet?).

2. I spoke with Dr. Turner, my sweet adviser. My previous quarterly meeting with Dr. Turner had been positive. He had told me how well I was doing on all my rotations and exams, and I had said I was doing just fine. I had looked good on paper, and I couldn't imagine how he might help. I did not catalogue the details of my day on the bridge, but told him I had been somewhat depressed. I figured Dr. Anderson had already told him about the day on the bridge. He murmured, "I've been there."

3. I visited our residency's counseling program on my own. I didn't find the counselor particularly helpful (granted, I only saw her for two sessions) and I didn't return.

4. After confiding in Jude about the bridge, I talked to her life coach/counselor one morning for almost two hours. He told me that since I had contemplated suicide so

sincerely, it would now forever remain as an option on my personal menu of "what to do in times of trouble." He told me to pay attention to my thoughts. It helped to talk to him.

5. My program director called me and instructed me to seek refuge in John and Jude, my sources of support. I took it as a hint to leave his faculty alone; that they had no business rescuing me from bridges and prescribing me antidepressants. He told me that he and Dr. Anderson would choose a primary care physician (PCP) for me — one outside the residency.

6. I saw the PCP. My visit was sad. I explained to her that I was exercising (I was running around the hospital and crying a lot), journaling (I had written... once?), was on Celexa and had an appointment set up with a therapist myself. I concluded there wasn't anything else to do. She agreed. It felt like we quietly sealed my coffin. She walked out. I sat, speechless for a few seconds, then followed her. I walked past her work station. She didn't look up at me as I left. I never felt so alone.

WHO I WAS NOW

I moved on to slightly less strenuous rotations. My mood didn't improve that much, but I settled into the routine of constant work. The panic and depression still followed me around, but I knew I wouldn't kill myself. I didn't deserve that way out; I had agreed to this training, and I was going to finish it.

I wanted to be a normal person. I wanted to be the supportive, creative, thoughtful partner to Jude I had been in the past. I had been a good listener. I had been excited to discuss life and all our plans and existential crises. I had prided myself on my attentiveness and had enjoyed going out, staying in, having a beer or talking over candlelight.

Now, I was just surviving.

I was desperate for sleep. I was desperate for Jude to not need me to listen. I was desperate to have one minute of time awake, alone, with enough mental clarity to grasp my life's purpose and remember what I was *doing*. My mind was a constant swirl, a revolving door of thoughts. One thought might be: *"Oh! That's right. I have been meaning to call him..."* And then another would intrude: *"Oh yes! I need to pay that bill..."* And then another: *"Right — her birthday is coming up..."* And then my pager would beep. And then 10 urgent emails would pop up about tasks due in 24 hours.

Sleep was empty. It swept by me and was never enough. I would awaken at the sound of my phone alarm and feel like I was emerging from a drugged stupor. I would wash my face and suit up for the day. I would stumble around, struggling to remember the basics.

What do I do next? Huh. Where are my shoes? Breakfast. Ugh. God, I can't eat. No, I have to eat. No real meal until I get home tonight.

Push bread into the toaster.

Close my eyes again.

OK, do I have my clothes on? Keys? White coat? Parking card? Stethoscope? OK. Where are my shoes?

POP! Goes the toaster.

Little things, like buttering toast, were much harder.

I felt brain-damaged.

And then, fifteen minutes later when I stepped foot into the hospital, a light shone on me. Or I changed my color like a chameleon. Or I put on a shield and my brain turned on. Choose a metaphor. I can't explain it. I was simply able to think more sharply. I felt tougher and suddenly was turned on mentally and physically, ready for war. I tackled the day with everything I had.

In the evening after we signed out, I left the hospital and walked to my car. My pace slowed back down to my semi-conscious self; back to that darker, duller, somewhat expressionless person. I drove home so extraordinarily exhausted so many days in residency that they run together now. I parked the car on our street. I collected my white coat, holding it from the collar to prevent all my precious papers from tumbling out. I grabbed my stethoscope and backpack, and zombie-walked into the apartment. Jude was always there to greet me with a warm attitude, candles, kind words and food.

She would ask about work. I usually could not answer her directly. I realized later, after graduation from residency, that my brain equated all questions with pimping, and that even the most innocent questions (i.e. 'What would you like for dinner?' or 'What movie would you like to see?') provoked terror or anger and immediately put me on the defensive. At the hospital, a question often meant I had done something wrong, and had better deliver the right answer – the one the questioner was thinking – quickly.

Jude did everything a wife could do to support me throughout residency. She tried to ease any extra worries from my life so I could concentrate on my work. She planned our time off so we could squeeze every last drop of relaxation out of it. She once packed my favorite sweatshirt, jeans, T-shirt and shoes and picked me up from work to go straight to an Indigo Girls concert. She cooked for me, came at a moment's notice to meet me, listened to me, and drove me to work when I needed it. She even visited me at the hospital while I was on call. We ate hot dogs in the cafeteria until I got an admission, and I left mine half-eaten.

I did my best under the circumstances. I helped around the house as much as I could. I made an effort to listen, encouraging her to talk about her day or share any thoughts. I made time to take walks with her and to have our date night once a week from 8 to 10 PM. I raced through sign-out to get home so we could eat together and be near each other until bed. I remembered her birthday and our anniversary. Somehow, by the end of the week, I always seemed to have put away the dishes, vacuumed, talked to my family, hung out with John and paid our bills.

I also went to her rehearsals and concerts — for her, for us, but mostly for myself. Her music kept me going.

Even so, there were many times I simply was not there for her.

In November of second year, Jude developed pneumonia. She was very sick, had a fever and was coughing constantly. One morning I was getting ready for work and she was coughing and crying, begging me to stay. I apologized and said I had to go to work, and walked out the door. I felt like a traitor.

In my third year, Jude was given a huge honor — she was asked to give a TEDx talk about her music. She asked me months in advance to come to the event, but I didn't know if I could; my rotation schedule hadn't been posted yet. Three weeks before the talk, I learned that I had to work that weekend. I asked 30 separate residents to cover for me, but no one was both willing and able to do it. So I worked while she experienced one of her most important moments. I had such remorse about not being there for her, after all the time she spent caring for me. I felt I had betrayed her.

WHAT I CAN FIT INTO A DAY

In my first year: Responding to around 25 emails. Making any number of patient phone calls. Refilling medications. Going to any number of meetings. Keeping patient logs. Reporting duty hours. Maintaining office hours. Typing many patient notes and completing several dictations. Ordering AM labs. Reading up on everything I don't know. Studying papers from the pharmacists. Catching up with surgeons after bouts of phone tag. Organizing a way for a kind, suicidal coworker to get appropriate help. Trying to find food. Rounding on my own personal patients. Completing rotation requirements. Giving personal medical advice to the nurses between other patients. Listening to the problems of my family and friends and offering – as cautiously as possible – medical advice. Performing some duty to prove I'm still committed to my relationship (e.g. put away the dishes and listen to a story about Jude's day).

In my second year — all of the above, plus: Checking intern orders. Teaching pre-med and medical students. Trying to keep up with current events. Applying and reapplying for vacation time. Breaking it to my family that I won't be home for Christmas — again. Listening for 10 minutes to a cardiologist in the hallway talk about his divorce, how stupid the ER is and how could his patient have seriously been deemed stable for transfer and why do his kids hate him and he's sick and has been working for 47 hours straight; he wonders if there is a connection and he wonders why are there no work-hour rules to protect attendings. Going back to another part of the hospital to complete a form the med student failed to fill out properly. Working against every fiber in my body that is saying:

Frances, you are a failure. You can't handle this. You are starving, about to pass out, incompetent, never deserved to go to med school in the first place. Your relationship is a mess, you never see your family and your clothes are disgusting. I bet you can't even remember the mechanism of action of aspirin. Your resume got you this far — but now you're doomed to either fail and get kicked out of the program or become a Terrible Doctor or get divorced or kill yourself.

NOTES ON ROTATIONS

The experiences on rotations were very different day to day, month to month. One month, I was in an operating room at Shadyside holding instruments and cutting where a surgeon told me to cut. The next, I was delivering babies at Magee. Then, I was working in Shadyside's Emergency Department, doing things such as admitting an 80-year-old woman who had come to the hospital for abdominal pain, only for us to find metastatic cancer throughout her abdomen. The next day, I was fielding questions on the phone about STDs and when to take a morning-after pill. The night after that, I might be sitting in a resident lounge in a hospital with three pagers, no other family medicine residents around, watching an episode of "Cops."

Family medicine is a collection of small and large insights into human life. We cut and sew skin, we diagnose disease, we keep checklists of immunizations, we comfort in times of confusion, we deliver babies and we take care of geriatric patients and their concerned families. A large portion of family medicine is dealing with psychological issues. I had suicidal and sometimes homicidal patients. I learned to keep myself between the patient and the door, for my own safety. I cared for patients with bipolar disorder, schizophrenia, delusional disorder, OCD, depression, anxiety and PTSD on a regular basis.

I involuntarily committed patients to WPIC, Pittsburgh's psychiatric hospital.

Over my pediatrics rotations, I worked in a newborn nursery, a pediatrician's office, Children's hospital and our family medicine clinic. I removed wax from tiny ears, taught new mothers about infant care, and ordered taper-down medicine regimens for drug-dependent newborns.

When I was on surgical rotations (both rural and urban), I stood like a statue for hours in operating rooms, cauterized stray bleeding vessels, and simultaneously fielded the surgeon's questions — which would range anywhere from, "What artery is this?" to "What does your father do for a living?" to "Are you married?" If I was feeling brave, I would admit that I was married, which always led to more questions. This meant I would be coming out to a roomful of techs and surgeons. Sometimes their reaction was relatively positive (something to briefly comment or joke about) and sometimes negative (no one would speak to me for the rest of the week). In the operating room, I would adjust my mask with my tongue and lips, scrunching my face to scratch little itches on my cheek. I would bend my legs up behind me one at a time, trying to keep them from locking or falling asleep. On breaks, I tried to be as useful as possible. I helped the staff transfer patients on and off the table, held doors, remembered to hold the catheters so they wouldn't get dislodged. When I couldn't figure out how to help, I sat in the locker room, reading up on relevant anatomy for the next case.

I worked in six different emergency departments throughout my medical training. There was a list of dozens of procedures I had to master over the three years of residency, so I had to be assertive to find opportunities to perform them. I cleaned wounds. I cut open abscesses and squeezed out the pus. An E.R. doc had me perform CPR on a dead patient and intubate him for practice. I talked to patients and scribbled down their stories. I found and provided vomit bins, sometimes too late. I was hit on by paramedics. I cared for a teenaged boy who had had multiple organ transplants and no arms or legs. I scrounged for signatures from attendings to get my hours signed off. I worked as efficiently as possible to make the machine of the hospital run smoothly, and to keep the patients, nurses and attendings happy.

JURY DUTY

In my second year, I received a jury duty notice in the mail and was instructed to report to the county courthouse in two weeks. I was to be on Floors that week, and fortunately I arranged (with help from Chief Orlando) for another resident to cover for me. The schedule on Floors is very strict — attendance is mandatory. Sort of like jury duty. Neither Jude nor I had ever had a summons, so I followed the rules I saw on the back of the card.

On the appointed day, I went to the courthouse. I filled out the paperwork I was given...

JUROR INFORMATION QUESTIONNAIRE
CONFIDENTIAL: NOT PUBLIC RECORD

LAST NAME _Southwick_   FIRST NAME _Frances_   MIDDLE INITIAL _M_

CITY/TOWNSHIP _Pittsburgh_

COMMUNITIES IN WHICH YOU RESIDED DURING THE PAST 10 YEARS ①_Weirton, WV_ ②_Lewisburg, WV_
③_Greeley, CO_ ④_Fort Collins, CO_

MARITAL STATUS: ☐ MARRIED ☒ SINGLE ☐ SEPARATED ☐ DIVORCED ☐ WIDOWED

OCCUPATION _Resident Doctor, Family medicine_ OCCUPATION(S) PAST 10 YEARS _medical student, desk clerk,_

SPOUSE/OTHER OCCUPATION _legally single, have partner, Judith Arus_ OCCUPATION(S) PAST 10 YEARS _pizza delivery_

NO. OF CHILDREN _Ø_ EDUCATION LEVEL: YOURS _BA, DO_ SPOUSE/OTHER _____ CHILDREN _____

RACE: ☒ WHITE ☐ AFRICAN-AMERICAN ☐ HISPANIC ☐ OTHER

		Yes	No
1.	Have you ever served as a juror before?...	☐	☒
	If so, were you ever on a hung jury?...	☐	☐
2.	Do you have any religious, moral, or ethical beliefs that would prevent you from sitting in judgment in a criminal case and rendering a fair verdict?..	☐	☒
3.	Do you have any physical or psychological disability that might interfere with or prevent you from serving as a juror?...	☐	☒
4.	Have you or anyone close to you ever been the victim of a crime?...	☒	☐
5.	Have you or anyone close to you ever been charged with, or arrested for, a crime other than a traffic violation?.....	☐	☒
6.	Have you or anyone close to you ever been an eyewitness to a crime, whether or not it ever came to court?..........	☐	☒
7.	Have you or anyone close to you ever worked in law enforcement or the justice system? This includes police, prosecutors, attorneys, detectives, security or prison guards, and court related agencies...........................	☐	☒
8.	Would you be *more* likely to believe the testimony of a police officer or any other law enforcement officer because of his or her job?...	☐	☒
9.	Would you be *less* likely to believe the testimony of a police officer or any other law enforcement officer because of his or her job?...	☐	☒
10.	Would you have any problem following the court's instruction that the defendant in a criminal case is presumed to be innocent unless and until proven guilty beyond a reasonable doubt?..	☐	☒
11.	Would you have any problem following the court's instruction that the defendant in a criminal case does not have to take the stand or present evidence, and it cannot be held against the defendant if he or she elects to remain silent or present no evidence?..	☐	☒
12.	Would you have any problem following the court's instruction in a criminal case that just because someone is arrested, it does not mean that the person is guilty of anything?...	☐	☒
13.	In general, would you have any problem following and applying the judge's instruction on the law?.................	☐	☒
14.	Would you have any problem during jury deliberations in a criminal case discussing the case fully but still making up your own mind?...	☐	☒
15.	Are you presently taking any medication that might interfere with or prevent you from serving as a juror?..........	☐	☒
16.	Is there any other reason you could not be a fair juror in a criminal case?.......................................	☐	☒

I hereby certify that the answers on this form are true and correct. I understand that false answers provided herein subject me to penalties under 18 PA.C.S. § 4904 relating to unsworn falsification to authorities.

SIGNATURE _~fr~ DO_   DATE _2/13/12_

WHITE-ORIGINAL   YELLOW-COPY   PINK-COPY   GOLD-COPY

…then was chosen as a juror on a criminal case (involving the sexual assault of a 6-year-old girl) and was told that I might have to be there for three additional days for the trial.

Panic set in. How would I get the rest of the dates covered? The judge's assistant explained that our employers would, by law, allow us off for these dates. The next 16 hours were complex. I called every resident in my batch to see if they could cover me. No one was available. I talked to Debbie Philips, and the program directors Dr. Hampton and Dr. Turner. They each asked why I hadn't pretended to be biased in my answers to the paperwork (in order to be excused from duty). I wasn't sure whether they were serious or not. They asked me to call the jury office and explain that my work involves patients who depend on my presence for their care. I spoke to an assistant to the judge who was presiding over my assigned case and told them this. I also pleaded with the juror coordinator (who I later learned was the judge's daughter, oddly) and explained my predicament.

Discussions related to jury duty really get under my skin. Many physicians told me that they never serve jury duty; they pretend to be biased or claim that their responsibilities are so great that they cannot serve. And I was strongly encouraged to do the same. I have always found it unfair that people in certain sectors of society are exempted from jury duty. I felt disgusted by the idea of using my "doctor card" to get out of what was my responsibility. The jury coordinator said she would talk to the judge, but she doubted she could help. I asked if they could talk to my boss, whom they insisted could not legally stop me from coming to the courthouse. I didn't know what to do. So

I went to work. I gave Dr. Hampton the number for the jury coordinator.

The jury coordinator called me after sign-out that morning.

"Ms. Southwick?" she said in an aggressive tone.

"Yes?"

"Judge says if you aren't at the courthouse at your appointed time, we will have men in uniform escort you to the courthouse."

My heart raced straight into my throat.

"I'll be there in 15 minutes."

I called Debbie Philips.

"If I don't go down there, they are coming for me," I said.

I had never been in trouble with the legal system and didn't want to be. I was torn between two government-funded institutions. But I was the one who would suffer the consequences from both sides. I felt helpless.

I whipped my Honda Fit into the $25 a day parking lot, got through security, then ran up the stone steps to the musty wood-paneled hallways to the jury room. I waited for the program director and the judge to sort it out.

As it turned out, the judge won. I served my time on the jury. My shifts were covered by my fellow residents.

As a member of the jury, my medical knowledge proved to be helpful. The perpetrator of the assault on the 6-year-old girl may have been found 'not guilty' had I not been there. I had to explain to the other jurors that no physical evidence would necessarily be visible, especially on a medical exam weeks after the crime. We convicted the defendant of all four counts against him. Afterward the judge confided to us that she believed he had committed the crime, and that we weren't allowed access to his past criminal records, which showed similar actions against the same victim in another state. The charges that we had convicted him of were the tip of the iceberg.

Serving on that jury was one of the proudest moments of my life. The plaintiff and her family had invested much time and energy, hoping for a just trial, and I was part of making a fair decision. The defendant had assaulted the girl repeatedly and almost got away with it. I wish other professionals would share my enthusiasm about jury service — it's just being a good citizen. On the other hand, the bias someone who doesn't want to serve is dangerous and could disrupt appropriate judicial decision-making.

Anyway, I think I did the right thing.

GOOD FACULTY

The Shadyside Family Medicine Residency faculty had a taxing job. They had to create doctors out of med school grads and be our role models without becoming our parents. Almost all of them took their jobs extremely seriously. When there was an opportunity for learning, the faculty seized it. Each had his/her own niche:

Dr. Davidson taught us the importance of writing effectively. The residents playfully made jokes about her for always correcting our notes and billing charges. I don't know if she had been assigned that task at a faculty meeting years ago, or if it was just her passion for detail. When we wrote a patient note that we knew she was going to approve, we called it a Davidson note, because it had to be perfect. I give her credit for helping me write appropriate and legally correct medical notes.

Dr. Cassidy taught us to remember to have fun. She came to every event, danced and drank with us, and brought her family along, too. She encouraged us to make our own decisions and learn from them.

Dr. Oxford gave us inspiration. He had been brought up in a family of doctors. I trusted him completely; I even recommended him to Jude for her medical care. He also was a family man and an accomplished harp player.

They also cared and involved us almost as family members. Dr. Hampton often invited all the residents and faculty to his home for home-cooked, organic dinners. Dr. Turner was very kind. Once, when I had a migraine, he called his wife and asked her to pick me up at the hospital (Jude was out of town). They let me take a nap at their house until I felt well enough to go home.

Our social science instructors were fantastic. We not only learned through lecture, anecdote, standardized patients and patient encounters; we also had Balint (a group for residents to confidentially discuss difficult patient encounters), and resident support group. It was such a comfort and relief to talk about challenging patient encounters and the difficulties of daily life in a nonjudgmental environment. We all enjoyed these sessions, and the stories we heard from each other helped us through many difficult days.

GOOD SENIORS

At one time, I was one of those pesky med students. I like to think I was slightly less annoying than a BCMS because I had more to learn and wasn't as cocky, but I was still a med student. While on my audition rotation at Shadyside (trying to woo the faculty and residents into ranking me highly for The Match), I was assigned to Floors. Dr. Hampton introduced me to Ernest, an intern who showed me around the hospital, pointing out where the shortcuts to different floors were and where to find the cafeteria. He also instructed me on how to find patients in the maze of Shadyside and how to write a decent note. Ernest was kind and thoughtful and his gestures were significant, making the experience quite enjoyable. His support helped me feel at home at Shadyside, and he was one of the main reasons I ranked the hospital as No. 1 in the Match.

As an intern, one Friday in clinic around 4 PM, I felt queasy. I still had two patients to see. I talked quickly with the first one, and really rushed the last one. My belly was gurgling loudly and I felt hot and lightheaded. I called Jude to come and get me. As soon as I entered the car, I reclined the seat back and curled up. At home I drew myself a bath and laid in the still water, shaking with chills, then exiting the tub with vomiting and diarrhea.

Orlando called to see how I was.

"Hey, Frances, just wanted to say we got you covered," he said. "Don't worry about call tomorrow. We'll see you Monday."

When Orlando heard I was sick, he tried to find someone to cover for me but wasn't successful. So he stepped in and took the 12-hour shift himself. He harbored no hard feelings. He simply took care of the problem at hand without making me feel guilty.

I was in a pretty low place at Magee Womens Hospital (clearly). Dr. Anderson arranged for me to talk with another resident, Joe Wooler, who had also had a very difficult month during his OB rotation as well.

"It sucks. It's terrible, right?" he said.

"I didn't know it was going to be this bad!" I said.

"I know. Everyone hates us. We don't know anything."

"The med students."

"The goddamn med students."

It was not the most positive meeting of the minds, but it was so satisfying to vent with an upper-classman about the challenges we faced. It made me feel a little less alone.

I was an intern on Floors. My senior resident paged me at 11 AM to assign me a new admission. So I began gathering data on the patient. As I was working on the admission form, another senior, Natalie, walked by.

"What are you doing?" she asked.

"New admission," I said, pointing to the paper.

"Seniors do admissions until noon. Everybody knows that," she said with a growl. And then she went to bat for me with the senior resident who had given me the assignment.

As I moved up the ranks, I tried to remember those lessons.

Be kind even when you are exhausted.

Try like hell to avoid abusing the people working under you.

Do what is right, even when it annoys someone.

DEATHS

I felt like I was living in another plane, because I was always so tired (there may be a theme, here). That constant fatigue led to a dream-like state that seemed as if my hospital/clinic world was the real world and all else was make-believe.

But life kept going on.

Heath and his wife, Jaime, were trying to have a baby. He had been going through a trying time: His dad was diagnosed with terminal cancer and then one of our (mostly his) psychotic patients had gone on a shooting rampage, killing and wounding innocent healthcare workers. Heath needed something positive in his life, and he and his wife were excited about the baby. They were choosing names. She miscarried. Then his dad went back into the hospital.

Another resident's father suddenly died and she had to leave. She had to beg her classmates to cover her mandatory rotation, knowing it would put a huge strain on her entire class.

These stressors, added to the already crushing pressure of residency, often seemed impossible to bear.

Jude and I had our own share of grief, too. Once the terror of the beginning of residency was over, we were presented with a mountain of grief.

Jude's father, then sister, then mother...all died.

Two of the calls woke us up; the other I received at work and had to tell Jude the news over the phone. The first death, her dad, happened in February of intern year. We knew it was coming — he had been in hospice for several months. I told my residency directors and chief residents that I would need time to attend the funeral. One director offered to front us some money for flights, which was kind, but I actually think it was strategic — to ensure that I would come back more quickly for work. We chose to drive.

The second death was in second year. It was her sister, Anne, who passed away at age 40. She had had heart problems for years, and died unexpectedly in her apartment; the cause was never elucidated. I had to call Jude from the office and tell her. Again, I made arrangements for my absence, and set up coverage for patient messages, my rotation, plus new nursing home duties. Then we flew to Colorado and organized Anne's funeral with her teenage children. It goes without saying that this was an extraordinarily difficult time for Jude. We worked hard to keep our lives going through the ordeal. I flew back to Pittsburgh two hours after the funeral to take call the next day.

The third death, her mom, was also unexpected and was the most difficult. It changed our lives. It left Jude partially incapacitated. She described her state of mind as "brain fog." She saw multiple counselors, because her original therapist (the one who told me to pay attention to my thoughts after my day on the bridge) had had a stroke during second year, rendering him aphasic. She just had to wait out her depression — it took about two years for her to feel like she could think clearly again.

GAINING CONFIDENCE

Small instances of learning occurred constantly. I absorbed immense amounts of knowledge without even thinking about it.

Late in second year, I began caring for a patient named Ms. Denver. Other residents in the office had seen her, but she was new to me. She was a small-framed woman who appeared even smaller by hunching forward and looking at the floor. Her eyes were welling up.

"How can I help you today?" I asked.

A long moment of silence followed.

Finally, she said, "No one is listening to me."

There was another long pause.

"My back hurts. My back always hurts. The medicine ain't working. My body is falling apart. I don't know what to do!"

She began crying now. I offered her a box of tissues, and she grabbed a few clumsily, wiping away her tears slowly. As I pieced together her medical history from old CT scans and notes and her personal account, something clicked. *Multiple arterial dissections? A valve replacement? Diffuse pains?*

"Ms. Denver, would you bend your finger back please?" I asked.

"What?"

"Just show me how far you can bend your finger back."

She bent her index finger and touched the back of her hand with it.

This clinched the diagnosis for me.

"I think I know what's going on," I said. "Just give me a few minutes."

I went to my work station and looked up Ehlers-Danlos Syndrome, a rare hereditary connective tissue disorder that causes very loose joints and skin, and sometimes heart and blood vessel problems.

I rushed to the attending who was supervising me and presented the case, explaining my idea.

"Mmmmm. Well, I don't know, Frances. A lot of really smart people have already been looking at this lady for years," he said skeptically.

I followed my hunch and sent her to a specialist and received confirmation of my diagnosis through genetic testing. Ms. Denver did in fact have Ehlers-Danlos Type 4, one of the most dangerous forms, which was splitting the insides of her blood vessels and causing pain all over her body. In the next few months, we discovered that her daughter also had the disorder.

It was my proudest diagnostic discovery. I was in the right place at the right time. When I was in medical school, I had had a practice case of a patient with Ehlers-Danlos, and it had stuck in my mind.

That case propelled me for months. What a high — to know I had figured out the missing link between this patient's complaints and the cause. This meant she had a diagnosis to explain all these strange medical problems and pains. Plus, a few treatment options were now available to help her live a bit longer and with less pain.

Ms. Denver is still a patient of mine today (along with many of her family members).

I never knew when moments like that would surface and reenergize me. I worked all the hours assigned to me and jumped through all the hoops, and occasionally there were beautiful moments such as those.

FUN FLOORS NIGHTS

There were good times in the hospital — especially at night. One week in third year, I was assigned to Floors Nights, 7 PM to 7 AM for five consecutive nights. I flew solo on the first night. Then I had Yoka, a hilariously fun, brand-new Japanese intern, as my intern for the next four nights.

Here are some notes from my journal that week:

Floors Night 1 of 5

Last night was the night of attendings' wives being admitted.

First up, a 63-year-old female patient of a prominent surgeon in the area admitted for unknown infection, quite sick. Her husband took the egregious liberty of putting in orders on her chart — maybe I would do the same thing for Jude. Who knows? I like him. He gifted me his "I like Obamacare" pin, which I put on the inside of my hoodie. I bet that would be grounds for dismissal if I were seen wearing it. I have a lot of respect for him; he once performed surgery on a patient of mine who no other surgeon would touch — a 30-something paralyzed female with a massive squamous cell carcinoma in her hip. He performed the daring feat of a hemipelvectomy (removing a leg and half a pelvis) on this lady, and somehow she survived. The last time I saw him, we were donating blood and childishly racing to fill our bags — he won by a landslide.

The second admission was pretty close to home — my own doctor's partner was admitted. It was one of the toughest admissions I have done in a while. I wanted to be helpful, supportive, caring and professional. I wanted to do it perfectly. But I barely passed for average as a resident on that case — missed a huge part of the diagnosis. Thank God I had to discuss that one with a scrupulous attending who caught my errors. Actually, she is one of the attendings with whom I always miss a piece of information or perform the physical examination too hurriedly or generalize the diagnosis in the presentation. Certain attendings just bring out my worst work, and I can't explain it.

Third was not really an admission — I received a page from an attending whose wife had been sick with belly pain all day, and he wanted to know who the Family Health Center attending was. I took a guilty sigh of relief — we had just capped (we only have to complete seven total admissions in each 12-hour period) until 7 AM, so I would be unable to do the admission. I was really shaken by that second case and wanted someone more objective to do the third admission. I hope that's what happened.

Now I am eating my first non-vegetarian meal since becoming a vegetarian three months ago: chicken-flavored Maruchan Instant Lunch (ramen noodles). There is something so comforting about hot water, in pretty much any form. I should be in bed — gotta get up in a few hours and pick up Jude at the airport! Hope her trip to Colorado wasn't too stressful...

Floors Night 2 of 5

Only two admissions but lots of teaching Yoka last night. Traveled around the hospital working with Yoka on her floor calls, teaching her about atrial fibrillation, hypotension, etc. At sign-out this morning, the attending pimped Yoka about her overnight patient management. She asked later if she had lost face for me. She hadn't.

I actually had four hours of sleep last night!

My young female patient with pancreatitis is improving and will have her gallbladder removed tomorrow. Thank god the scan was wrong; there was no mass in her pancreas — just inflammation.

Now, off to vote — Obama versus Romney. Ryan the intern asked us if he could "exercise his right to vote" — nice use of distancing language to try to get an unemotional, affirmative response. I used the same language for my jury duty last year — I was carrying out my "civic duty."

Floors Night 3 of 5

Obama won for his second term.

No admissions overnight — I guess everybody was glued to their TVs.

We did have a couple of floor calls, though. Natalie's (first year as an attending!) patient, who has end-stage COPD and gets admitted for severe shortness of breath fairly frequently, was screaming at her nurses that she couldn't breathe. Yoka and I hiked up to the floor and found the patient demented and hollering at her young nurse who was standing nervously in the doorway.

"Hiya Ms. K!" I called.

"I can't breathe! Someone's gotta do something!" she bellowed.

Immediately I was pleased by her ability to stay conscious and answer so loudly. She was stable but very anxious, which certainly worsens the sensation of breathlessness when one is having trouble taking in air.

Yoka and I moved to the patient's bedside. Her TV was blaring about the election. Ms. K's oxygen saturation was 94 percent on 4 liters of oxygen. She thought it was 2002.

Our task was to ensure that the patient was comfortable. We administered a tiny dose of olanzapine ODT (antipsychotic med that disintegrates in the mouth) and my favorite part of the treatment regime — I changed the channel to Lifetime.

We didn't get any further calls about Ms. K.

Floors Night 4 of 5

My pre-med student showed up today unannounced after not showing up for three of our previous shadowing dates. I politely asked her to leave and to be more professional with her next shadowing experience. My team now thinks I am a huge badass.

I have learned more Japanese (from Yoka) the last three nights than medicine, that's for sure. Arigato (thank you). Do itashi mashita (you're welcome). I am having that feeling of making a friend again — it has been so long.

Last night Yoka and my snacks were: Simply Naked Pita Chips, Laffy Taffy (left over from zero trick-or-treaters to our apartment this year), sweet gooey stuff from some other country, a lemon bar, a banana, roasted vegetables.

Jude's Facebook page has become honey to her swarm of passionate friends — why the country will be going to go to hell in a hand basket or be saved from evil tyranny since Obama was reelected. She is celebrating and some of her friends are... not.

Floors Night 5 of 5

The final night, we capped in the first two hours; all seven admissions before 8:45. Four for me, three for Yoka, with me supervising.

Here's how the last 30 hours went down:

6:30 PM	suited up in my boots, green khaki pants, white Hanes T-shirt with pale-blue scrub-top, single pocket filled with important numbers and old Palm Pilot, drove in old Subaru to work
7:00 PM	signed in with Ryan, Yoka; handed out chocolate chip anddecaf espresso cookies Jude made for the team
7:17 PM	took group photo to commemorate my final Floors shift and started first two admissions: PID (pelvic inflammatory disease) and chest pain.
7:26 PM	called with third admission: RUE (right upper extremity) weakness/numbness.
7:30 PM	called with fourth admission: chest pain with history of PE/DVT (blood clots in lung and leg)
7:42 PM	called with fifth and sixth admissions: chest pain with history of anomalous coronary artery (abnormal anatomy of the blood vessels to the heart) and cellulitis (skin infection)
8:44 PM	called with seventh admission: asthma exacerbation; also caught up talking to attendings, writing orders and dictating notes on all the admissions
3:00 AM	had heart-to-heart with intern Yoka, worked more on dictations/orders/notes

5:10 AM	took a nap
6:30 AM	saw patient with pancreatitis, completed discharge paperwork
7:00 AM	signed out
7:30 AM	saw patient with history of PE, DVT (blood clots in lungs/legs) with chest pain
8:10 AM	wrote discharge summary on patient, said goodbye and well done to Yoka
8:40 AM	handed out remainder of cookies to my favorite nurses and HUCs (health unit coordinators, who are essentially the office managers of the hospital floors)
8:50 AM	walked to clinic
9:00 AM	saw first of seven patients at the clinic (the eighth was a no-show)
12:35 PM	completed seeing patients
1:00 PM	faxed details to charity care organization for patient with newly-diagnosed HIV to get his new meds
1:30 PM	took care of patient phone messages, patient paperwork for FMLA (Family Medical Leave Act), oxygen, physical therapy, etc.
2:00 PM	called Jude on way home, realized I hadn't eaten since before work previous night
2:30 PM	kissed Jude hello (no hugs — wearing overnight scrubs)
2:35 PM	ate lunch
3:30 PM	took a nap
7:30 PM	woke up; listened to Jude's new album with The Early Mays — so perfect
8:00 PM	ate dinner — nachos a la Jude — and watched a movie on Netflix
10:00 PM	YouTube surfing with Jude

10:35 PM	wrote this entry
11:00 PM	showered
11:20 PM	did some stretching and then went to bed

I'm looking forward to being an attending. But I will also be leaving a team. I won't be in the struggle anymore. On the other hand, having a saner, less-hectic schedule means I will hopefully be a healthier and happier person.

HEATH

By the time I was a senior resident, I was stronger. I had learned to handle things. Intern year had beaten the hell out of me, and I had climbed my way back up the ladder, past my former self, and felt like I was starting to belong. Or at least I knew how to survive.

One Saturday evening, I arrived at Three East to sign in for a night shift. I greeted the nurses and aides with a wide grin, as this was to be my 104th call shift over two years — my final in-house (in-hospital) call...*forever*. In the morning, July 1st, I would sign out to a fresh team, including two brand-new interns.

That night, as I had done for the last two years, I began the shift by taking a blank sheet of paper from the printer and folding it lengthwise, labeling one half "calls," the other "to do." I joked around with Adam, my intern for the evening. He was describing a new cream he was using to cure the red, flaky skin that had developed on his face. He was thinner than he had been at the beginning of the year. He was pale. He seemed anxious; his eyes darted around the room. Nonetheless, Adam did a pretty good job of concealing his depression with banter, laughter and playing string quartets for us on his iPhone. As we talked, my phone buzzed in my pocket.

"Int Heath" was calling. (All my former classmates are to this day listed in my phone as "Int," short for intern, because I saved all of their numbers in Orientation Week.)

This was odd — Heath had called me perhaps three times *ever*, always to quickly sign out patient information. I glanced at the Board — there were no Heath patients. He was supervising the interns over the past week, but would have no reason to call me about their patients. I answered casually.

"Hey man, what's up?"

"Hey dude, it's Heath. What's goin' on?" His voice had a hint of worry.

"Nothin'. I have the last call so we were just getting ready to sign out. What's goin' on with you?" I said.

"Uh...just...I don't know. You got a second?"

Now he had my full attention. I headed toward the stairwell for some privacy.

"Yeah man, of course. No admissions pending. What's goin' on?"

I softened my tone from what Jude calls my FBC (football coach) voice to something between concerned friend and confident physician.

"I'm just — I don't know," he said. "I'm going through some transitions right now. I'm pacing around my house. I...I just wanted to tell you that I love you and Jude, and I think you're awesome. I'm not a bigot, and I want you to know that. I just...I don't want you to think I'm an asshole."

His voice was cracking, like someone on the edge. I coaxed him to continue talking. He explained that he had been undergoing intensive outpatient therapy three times a week, and he had to curtail his sessions for the past month because he was on Floors. He reminded me of his stressors — dad dying of cancer, wife suffering a miscarriage, our psychotic patient killing and wounding people in the lobby of WPIC. Heath had worked for months to help this patient get the appropriate treatment and this event was still devastating for him.

I asked more about the therapy — was it helping?

"Yeah, I think so, I mean I started the intensive three-day-a-week therapy because I had… um…tried stuff."

I broke out in a sweat as I flashed back to my intern year, recalling my day on the bridge. We ended our conversation with a plan. He said he would play video games and wait for his wife to come home from work. I called his adviser, who then contacted Heath and called me back, assuring me he would be all right, that the department would address the issue. I still felt unsettled by the phone call, but completed my work and headed home.

That night, Jude asked me sleepily, "Do you still like me?"

"I love you."

"Miss my mom," she said softly.

I petted her hair and tried to present myself as a calm partner. But my mind was in a state of turmoil — worried about my pending notes, my pending patient calls, Heath, getting sleep, maintaining my weight, how to work faster in the office, my current rotation, how to learn enough and please the attendings enough to pass the rotations, how to get more procedures done so I could graduate on time, and a thousand other concerns that swirled together into a haze…

I closed my eyes tight and took a slow, measured breath. I was a third year resident, now. The home stretch. I forced myself to relax for a minute. For Jude.

Two weeks later, when I was in the office waiting for my 4 PM patient to arrive, Angela rushed into the cubicle (previously a supply closet) where we worked on notes.

"Frances, I want to talk to you about something," she said, her voice grave with concern. I had never seen her so troubled. I shut the door.

"What's goin' on?" I asked.

"It's about Heath. He called me yesterday."

I remembered my uneasy conversation with him about his depression.

Angela explained that she had been at the office, working the evening shift, when Heath phoned her, sounding very upset. He told her that he didn't know what he was going to do, apologized for his behavior, and could she please not think he was an asshole. The conversation was similar to the one I had had with him.

"He had obviously been drinking," she said. "He kept saying things like, 'Angela, I can't take this anymore. I put on a happy face for everybody, but I'm not happy. I used to be. I'm so depressed.'"

Then things escalated.

"He told me he had a gun. He said, 'I'm going to eat this bullet. I can't take it. I have the gun right here in my hand.'"

Angela said that she tried everything to keep him talking on the phone. She even appealed to his sense of guilt, by saying,

"You wouldn't do that to me, would you?" She called one of our attendings and an emergency contact line. She got in her car and tried to find his house but got lost. Finally, when she arrived at his place, police were in the driveway and they were taking Heath to the hospital. He was drunk and had injured his hand by punching through a wall.

A few nights later, Jude talked with Heath's wife, Jaime, for about an hour. More details of Heath's life came out. I had wondered for some time if Heath had a drinking problem and indeed this was the case; his alcohol use had skyrocketed as a coping strategy for the stress of residency.

While Heath was healing up for a few weeks in his hometown, we all covered for him at the hospital. He came back, stuck it out and worked his way through the rest of the year. He also joined AA. It was rocky, and he had to work through many issues, but he did it.

Life stressors like sick relatives, deaths and psychotic/dying/angry/drug-seeking patients are difficult. But when you couple them with the time and energy constraints of residency, they can seem insurmountable. Even the toughest get pulled down. It takes a team to keep each member afloat.

UBIQUITOUS

Heath and I weren't the only ones who had difficulties. Almost everyone I knew on the road to doctorhood either had a breakdown or dropped out. Many had thoughts of, or made attempts at, suicide — and a few, unfortunately, succeeded.

The difficult pre-med years produced the most dropouts, weeding out those who were not 100 percent committed to medicine from the get-go. They found the prerequisite classes (nicknamed, literally, "weed-out" classes) too challenging, or couldn't get the hang of the MCAT, or they found the process was too tedious or expensive. There were also students who gave up after an initial med school non-acceptance year.

After admission to medical school, there was much less wiggle room for dropping out. Most (certainly not all) of those who start med school became full-on physicians. But through much hardship. The students who had problems with academics but squeaked into med school by some miracle really struggled. The learning process there is often compared to attempting to drink from a fire hose. It was hard, but most students who got that far were there because they could handle it. The 90 percent of us who passed the first year were fairly locked in; the cost of each year of medical school is between $30,000 and $55,000. We invested many years, tears and dollars in the process of becoming a doctor, so most of us found a way to stick with it. Even for those few students *without* the loan handcuffs, some were still under pressure to stay put — because of military or scholarship obligations or family expectations. Most of us didn't have much of a Plan B. There was enormous pressure to stay the course. So most of us kept pushing, even when it was hurting us.

There were exceptions.

Some failed the Boards. One friend of mine, Rhiannon, was an avid studier. She spent hours in the library, highlighted her notes and never missed a class. She also was very personable and approachable. But she couldn't pass the Boards. WVSOM allowed her three or four attempts, and then gave her the boot. So, with over $200,000 of debt (plus undergraduate loans, I assume), she was on her own, in search of a new career. Even the student with the highest GPA in our med school nearly failed the Boards due to anxiety.

Med school is tough, but *residency* brings an eclipsing level of stress. Two weeks after graduating from residency, a close friend told me, "I feel like I just got out of prison." Each year of the residency process has its unique challenges. Intern year is toughest for those afraid of looking stupid; that is an intern's job – to continually be asked questions in front of her peers and oftentimes look stupid. Second year is hard for those who are afraid of being in charge; they are now 'senior' residents, supervising interns. Third year is most difficult for residents who have a hard time making life decisions; this is when residents decide where to live permanently, which job to take, etc.

And the first year after residency is terrifying for physicians who are uncomfortable making diagnosis and treatment plans independently; no attending is there to back them up.

Nikki (our extra-bubbly intern classmate) was bright but couldn't quite catch on to a few concepts necessary for advancement to second year. She had to repeat part of intern year, which was a big blow to her spirit. I didn't see her smile for a year or so.

Arianna was single and lived alone. She invited Jude and me over for her birthday, and we found that her refrigerator was broken. Arianna was still eating milk products and meat she stored in the lukewarm temperature, because she simply had no time to have it repaired. The three of us shared some questionable drippy birthday cheesecake in her unkempt apartment.

Maria started her intern year wearing flawless makeup and perfect hair. This may sound superficial, but her appearance was a strong part of her identity; she referred to herself as a fashionista. It must have taken an hour and a half for her to get ready each morning. By the end of her intern year, I barely recognized her. She was pasty and sullen, devoid of cosmetics, wearing smelly scrubs like the rest of us. Personality whittling is inevitable; there is just not enough time to keep oneself whole.

Wayne started internship as a nice caring guy and turned into the nastiest resident I knew. He felt his work would never be as good as it needed to be, so he gave up. He drank heavily at residency get-togethers and took his aggression out on everyone, making cruel jokes about patients and physicians.

Angela wept in the stairwell to me (in third year) that she was really losing it, even losing faith, afraid to pray.

John's relationship with Matt crumbled over the course of residency. They didn't spend enough time together, which eventually led to infidelity and a messy split. As I am, he is now working through issues pushed under the rug through the years of med school and residency.

Jessie, a surgical resident friend, attempted suicide. I remember bumping into her in the parking lot at Magee.

"Hey! How are you?" I asked.

"Oh, just leaving."

"Nice! You on call?"

"Yeah." She then told me that the night before she had put a plastic bag over her head in an attempt to suffocate herself.

"I thought I could figure it out but I can't," she said. "Do you know any good therapists?"

Once trained, we must find our way through life after residency. We have to find a job that isn't going to *keep* us miserable. Many of us find this a difficult task. We are so accustomed to our horrible schedules that we blindly accept an equally horrible schedule, just with better pay.

Dr. Mumford, one of WVSOM's brilliant anatomists, was previously a surgeon who changed his career because of the "stress of the surgeon's lifestyle." After two years of teaching us, and years of antidepressants and electroconvulsive therapy for his severe depression, he committed suicide.

Edith was two years ahead of me in school. I remember her partner, Bobbi, telling us stories about Edith's intern year, when she considered dropping out to join the police force. She was also hoping that she'd be in a car accident on the way to or from work, as a way out. While I was a medical student,

Edith encouraged me to reconsider my choice of career, to find another field before entering residency.

"Don't do it, Frances. Really. I wish I hadn't."

If you could go back in time and watch people boarding the Titanic, would you scream at them to turn back, or would you watch them and wave, knowing that they would ignore your warnings? There were some survivors, weren't there?

After one particularly hard day, I could barely form sentences when I spoke to my mom on the phone. I was brain-dead, and very sad. She told me a story about a cardiologist neighbor of hers who (many years prior) had come home after a month of internship, calling in sick for the following day. He drove to the U.S. National Parks Service and applied to be a ranger. He was turned down because he was overqualified and was forced to go back to the hospital.

Diana Brown, a former classmate of Jude's, had a brother who was a doctor. He quit his family medicine program four months prior to graduation because he couldn't handle the stress, and moved into Diana's basement, unemployed.

On my interview day at St. Margaret's (fourth year of med school), I noticed a plaque with the name of a former resident. Later in the day, I asked the program director how many residents had started the program and not graduated. He looked through his lists of residents from the last five years. His eye caught the same name as the one on the plaque. He told me that this one had not made it. He had ended his life in his intern year.

In my two complimentary UPMC counseling sessions after the bridge incident, my counselor said she simply wished we residents could talk to each other more. Our stories of shame, guilt, desperation and depression were all very similar. I wondered how many residents had come through that office.

After finishing residency, I learned that two UPMC anesthesia physicians – one resident, and one attending – had committed suicide *while* I was a resident at UPMC Shadyside. And I never knew. It was kept private to 'protect the families.'

Secrecy begets secrecy, which begets shame. Physicians feel they need to be the strongest ones in the room, at all times. So they put on a tough exterior or a permanent smile at work. And then no other doctors know their pain. How can physicians survive without knowing how much the other physicians are suffering?

Then from the handbook we were given for life after residency (given to us in third year), I learned a few statistics: Those who work 50-plus hours a week are three times more at risk of developing an alcohol-abuse problem. According to Inc. magazine, "20 [consecutive] hours without sleep is equal to a 0.1 blood alcohol level. That is equivalent to five or six drinks." More interestingly, the suicide rate for doctors is higher than in any other profession. The trouble seems to disproportionately affect female physicians, who have suicide rates four times higher than any other professionals. Only 26 percent of female doctors report being very satisfied with their medical practices. 15 percent of all doctors will be unable to perform their professional responsibilities at some point in their career because of mental illness, alcoholism or drug dependency. And remember, these are high functioning overachievers. These are the people who can make things work. The people you trusted in high school, college and now to take care of you and your family. (Skertich, 2010)

PIZZA AND WHISKEY

By the very end of third year, Jude and I were fried. Most of her family were dead, and my spirit was crushed; I didn't know who I was anymore. We were sick of ourselves and of each other. We didn't know whether it was better to be near or to avoid each other.

I sat in the living room, melting into our second-hand couch. Jude stood in the kitchen, stunned, weeping. We both felt empty and lonely, with a sort of passive fury, too exhausted to make an effort.

My mind wandered. I thought about John, who was at my graduation party the night before. He had been reminiscing about our college days when tears began to well up in his eyes. He looked as lost as I felt.

I thought about Heath and his wife. Would they make it?

I also thought about my new job that would start in a month. Would it be a reprieve?

"*Blee-ee. Blee-ee. Blee-ee,*" the oven chirped that it was ready for work. It was pizza night. We had no energy for cooking.

Jude walked into the dining room. Her hair was frizzy and unkempt, and she wore an old pair of jeans and a holey white T- shirt. Her eyelids were purplish from crying, but it made her look so beautiful. I always felt a little guilty about thinking so.

I sliced pizza, putting one half of the pie on each plate — so we wouldn't have to waste energy getting up for seconds. I walked to the living room with dinner. Jude put on an episode of "Cheers" on Netflix for dinner entertainment. We watched without speaking.

When we were finished eating, we stared at each other.

"I don't have anything left," Jude whispered.

I nodded. We both were moving in slow motion.

I reached my hand out, and touched her thigh.

"I think I need a drink," I said.

I went to the kitchen and brought back two jelly glasses and a bottle of Maker's Mark. I poured myself enough for more than a buzz.

Generally, Jude does not drink. My parents always try to get her to drink, because that's my family's way of saying, "Relax! We love you!" Her friends try to get her to drink so they feel better about drinking. I always offer when I have one because I think it's polite, but she always refuses. She grew up with a stepdad who loved his Jack Daniel's, and she says that the years with him turned her off to alcohol. She didn't even have a drink at our wedding.

I motioned to the other glass as a question, and Jude nodded, her face twisted up with tears. I poured her one to match mine.

I smoothed her hair over her left ear and wiped her tears. She closed her eyes and pushed her forehead into my hand, soothing herself like a cat. We finished up our glasses of whiskey with a shudder, and then crawled to the floor. We laid motionless for half an hour or so. I nuzzled my head in the crook of her neck, and we both wept.

At least we still had each other.

THE MOST IMPORTANT CHAPTER

My friends and family get angry when I tell them these stories. They demand to know what can be done about the problem of depression in the medical field, and in particular, the high rate of suicide over the course of the training process. Burnout in the medical field is extremely high; about half of all doctors are classified as having burnout (Peckham, 2015) (defined as loss of enthusiasm for work, feelings of cynicism, and a low sense of personal accomplishment). The specialties with the highest percentage of burned out physicians are critical care, emergency medicine, family medicine, internal medicine and surgery.

Why do so many doctors want to kill themselves?
...and...
Does it have to be this hard?

PROBLEMS

1. **Information explosion.** The fact is that today's doctors in training are bombarded with an impossible amount of information which they must master in order to become competent professionals. The medical knowledge that a physician in 1950 was required to learn is much different from what doctors in 2015 need to absorb. Over the last few decades, technology has changed drastically, and as such, so has our understanding of the human body

and pathology. Medical information is constantly shifting and evolving. There is now a rising sea of medicines we must understand and prescribe. Keeping up with all these new developments by reading the latest literature — especially on pathophysiology and pharmacology — is overwhelming for even the brightest physicians.

2. **Exhaustion.** I know that I came up against many challenges during rotations in med school — and felt vulnerable as a result — but I still had hope, and had some time to process. I took refreshing walks. I had enough time after work hours to research the questions I had formed about patients throughout the day. But the frenzied years of residency do not offer many breaks to refocus. And after residency, it often does not improve. There are no work-hour rules for attending physicians, so the sky is the limit.

3. **Too many requirements to fit into three short years.** To accommodate the 80-hour work week, today's residents simply take the work home to avoid breaking the rules. At the end of each week, residents must report their hours electronically, detailing the work done each day. Residents must fill out evaluations of every rotation, every resident and every attending with whom they work. Residents are also required to do scholarly work. In our program, this took the form of Quality Improvement projects, wherein each resident must envision a way to improve patient care, then research and prepare the change, carry it out, study the results, and give four lectures to the faculty and fellow residents over the three years. All of this work is done in the resident's "own time." Residents are required to participate in journal club each year, wherein they review and present their professional opinions of a medical journal article. They

prepare and give mini-lectures to fellow residents and medical students on rotations (such as Floors — imagine fitting that into the schedule). They take Boards *twice* in residency: once in intern year and once in third year. Aside from Boards, each year they also take half-day exams, to determine their strengths and weaknesses. Over the three-year period, residents must master dozens of procedures, and for each of these skills must seek independent evaluation from a supervising doctor. This is not to mention the old tasks that remain — family medicine residents must be on call constantly in case one of their pregnant patients goes into labor. Family medicine residents must have 1,650 outpatient visits by the time they graduate. Residents must participate in the recruitment new interns (travel to fairs and medical schools to sell the residency program), attend hours-long dinners with recruits, and give them tours of the hospital between other duties (recruitment dinners are not counted as work hours). Between their other daily tasks, residents also must teach pre-med and medical students. This is not paid. Much of the training of medical students falls on residents. During third year, residents must (while still completing all other requirements) find a house and a job (this includes interviewing, sometimes across the country).

SOLUTIONS ALREADY IN PROGRESS

The good news is – we can change! And we are changing! We don't have to continue to suffer in the old dogma. We can accept that medicine and the role of the family doctor has changed in this country.

In recent years there have been many positive changes in medical training, including standardization of residency curriculum, higher standards of education and multiple layers of supervision to decrease the risk of inexperienced physicians making bad choices in a hospital alone at night. Balint (in which our residency participated) is a discussion group led by mental health professionals that (which we were able to attend about ½ the time due to scheduling/location details) helps physicians rekindle empathy and express their emotions about challenging patient situations. This program could easily be extended to every US residency program, giving residents a structured forum, at least for their patient-related difficulties. We also had two designated times (20 minutes of support group three times a month and, in first year only, four hours of "intern night" once a month) to process our experiences with one another.

There seems to be more focus on compassion in medicine today, especially in family medicine. Residents are taught from the beginning to remember the patient and his/her values as central to each encounter.

Residents also get vacation days — a relatively new concept; previously, residents would get together secretly and agree on which days they would plan to call in sick.

These changes are well-meaning. My training in family medicine was excellent, but the residents there still feel the same desperation that their predecessors did in The House of God. I work with them a week out of every month, and watch as they gain and lose dozens of pounds, cry in stairwells, and take unplanned breaks for mental and physical illnesses. But mostly, I watch them take excellent care of patients and try to prove that they are strong and smart. They don't want anyone, especially us attendings, to know how much they are suffering.

NEW IDEAS FOR SOLUTIONS

1. **Ensure that pre-med students know what they are getting into.** I was able to work with three pre-med students from Carnegie Melon University over the course of my residency years. This, I believe, was a valuable experience for those students. Residents are perfectly suited to tell pre-med students about life in medicine. Currently, pre-med students often shadow attending physicians for four hours (total!), but they are not usually exposed to residents. Pre-med students need to know what the life of a resident is like.

2. **The NBME and NBOME need to enforce standardization of the clinical years of medical school.** I was clearly unprepared for Children's and Magee Womens rotations. The despair I felt was not due to a single problem, but the culmination of issues. I was in a new and sometimes hostile environment, I felt overwhelmed and the hours were intense. I started each of these rotations exhausted. But I could have handled the stress better if I had been more prepared. Many medical schools require their students to complete "Shelf Exams" prepared by the NBME (National Board of Medical Examiners). Med students take a Shelf Exam at the end of each clinical rotation. These ensure standardization of knowledge gained during clinical rotations. But not every medical school requires its students to take Shelf Exams; mine did not. Even though I had been a good student, I did not get all the information I needed; my clinical experience was piece-meal. I am not suggesting that Shelf Exams are the only way to standardize the learning, I am saying that medical schools and their governing bodies need to take more responsibility for ensuring that their medical students are adequately prepared for residency.

3. **Pay the physicians who train medical students.** The physicians who train medical students in the clinical years (years three and four) are sometimes *not paid*. This boggles my mind. These instructors volunteer their time to help train upcoming doctors. What incentive did they have to train me well, other than their kind hearts?

4. **Medical schools and residency programs need to provide mental health care to medical students and residents.** Every physician, when looking back, shudders about some step in the training process. Any physician can easily remember which year (almost always during residency) was the worst. Outside the challenges I have outlined, each step of the training process holds its own unique difficulties. Medical school is difficult for those who have weaknesses in academics or test taking anxiety. The clinical years of medical school and intern year are difficult for those who are afraid of appearing incompetent. The second year of residency is hard for those who are afraid of a leadership role. The third year challenges those afraid of finally cutting the apron strings after being students for 30 years, and becoming independently functioning physicians. Sadly, most students and residents don't know their own weaknesses until they are flailing. To identify and assist those who are struggling at each step (and there are always people struggling at each step), I believe trainees need mandatory meetings with therapists at least quarterly. Medical students and residents are often quite stoic, wanting to impress faculty and attendings with their ability to stay late, take on more than the average resident, and be the smartest in the group. They are usually perfectionists, and will use any means possible to hide their weaknesses. This must be addressed head on. In addition, those with a history of depression or substance abuse need further

specialized treatment to help reduce the risk of and monitor for relapse.

5. **The RRC (Residency Review Committee, part of the Accreditation Council for Graduate Medical Education) could better optimize family medicine residency curriculum requirements.** The amount of work a family medicine resident is expected to squeeze into three years is not realistic. The curriculum of those three years is extraordinarily important. There are many ways family medicine residency training could be more effective. I believe that there should be much less focus on both obstetrics and surgery in family medicine training; much of this training is irrelevant for the current family doctor. Restructuring the curriculum would allow for fewer hours per shift during the other rotations, thereby reducing stress and sleep deprivation.

    a. **Firstly, most family doctors are not delivering babies.** According to the American Academy of Family Physicians, only *"fifteen percent* of AAFP members report delivering babies, and those members delivered 20 babies on average in 2012."* (AAFP, 2015) One might ask, "Isn't it the legacy of the family physician to deliver babies as part of their practice?" Yes, it once was, but that is quickly changing. Why? Because of the enormous legal risk. Because the amount of time and energy spent on obstetrical call, in addition to the other work of a family doctor, is overwhelming. Because the malpractice insurance is extremely expensive. Because obstetrics stands alone as its own entire, complex specialty. The faculty, residents and nurses at Magee Womens Hospital were not mean-spirited people out to get me; I was simply another family medicine resident who was ill-prepared, and they were annoyed to have to deal with the repercussions. The idea that family docs can be proficient in modern obstetrics after a mere 40 deliveries over eight weeks of training, is, to be frank, absurd. Those family medicine doctors who choose to deliver should be granted the right to do so, but need more training, such as an obstetrical fellowship for family doctors (these already exist!).

b. Secondly, family doctors are not surgeons, anymore – so they don't need much surgical training. On one of my surgical rotations in residency, the surgeon rolled his eyes and said to me, "I don't know why they have you guys do this rotation. I don't know what to teach you. You aren't going to be a surgeon!" He was right. Today, family doctors generally perform minor office procedures (draining abscesses, cleaning wounds, freezing warts and performing mole removals), but nothing that would require anesthesia or an operating room. Surprisingly, eight weeks of training in family medicine residency training is devoted to surgical rotations, during which family medicine residents stand painfully in operating rooms, trimming sutures, and learning next to nothing that will be relevant to their practices. These hours spent in surgery could be significantly reduced or eliminated.

6. **Be kind to outsiders.** Isn't it sad that no Shadyside resident before my class received an intern survival guide at Children's? This was such a simple oversight, yet family medicine residents for years had been struggling through this Children's rotation without the appropriate guidebook. Were residents who came before me simply afraid to speak out? Or did they not know the book was in existence? Either way, there should have been a fix to this problem before it ever became a problem. Hospitals with visiting residents need to make a special effort to include residents who are from other hospitals. Learning a hospital system is a very complex process, and outsiders need special attention.

7. **Speak up if you see a problem, and respect those who ask questions.** Residents are often nervous to bring up problems. I was often too scared to ask questions, because I wanted to maintain my appearance as a smart new doctor. I didn't want to let my guard down or let anyone know I had knowledge gaps. This is dangerous. Fortunately, the culture at Shadyside was usually open and amicable, such that residents were usually able to respectfully voice their concerns without fear of repercussions. But this is not always the case. Many residency programs do not foster an atmosphere of camaraderie. This is paramount for residents to learn appropriately, avoid potentially dangerous medical errors, and to make the system better for everyone. This is particularly difficult for many IMGs. The culture of medicine in many countries is extremely hierarchical. If one is a student or resident, one always defers to one's superior, and never questions authority. Asking questions is an essential part of learning. Open communication should be encouraged not only between residents and attendings, but among nurses, patients, respiratory technicians,

transport staff...everyone. All must work together to provide safe care and ensure every team member is able to comfortably ask questions.

8. **Reduce bureaucracy, where possible.** In a 2015 report on physician burnout, "too many bureaucratic tasks" was the main complaint of physicians. (Peckham, 2015) Physicians must follow the guidelines of so many different governing bodies, they often feel that decision making is out of their hands. Physicians need autonomy to be able to practice medicine happily and well. Varying insurance rules, varying drug costs, difficulties obtaining medical records from outside laboratories and hospitals, demanding hospital administration, countless measures of performance, fear of litigation – these are all realities of the modern American medical system. Rules about the tedium of how to order even simple tests change frequently. Wise leadership in healthcare administration is direly needed. A single payer system and a national electronic health record would dramatically reduce the stress and guesswork physicians are constantly forced to endure.

APPENDIX A: WHAT I MISS ABOUT RESIDENCY

1. Sneaking in afternoon talks with Dr. Turner, my adviser. I would wander by his office now and then to see if he could spare a minute. I found it comforting to speak with someone who was empathetic, yet grounded enough not to focus only on the negative side of residency.

2. Texting with Dr. Oxford about what to watch on Netflix.

3. Being on call with sleep-deprived, funny residents. We didn't pick who we were on call with; it was a random assignment. When we were matched with a compatible call companion, the shift had bright spots and laughter.

4. Savoring my one day off. Jude and I became experts at this. We could strategize a miniature retreat into a single 24-hour period.

5. Intern's Night. Once a month for four hours, interns spent time together, sharing stories, laughing, hugging and playing. I wish we would have continued the tradition after intern year.

6. Caring faculty. Our bosses were personable and approachable, and we used them as examples to carry us through tough times. We knew they had families and

hobbies and they seemed pretty happy. They were living, breathing goals.

7. Stripping off disgusting clothes and taking a blazing hot shower after a delivery.

8. Learning random awesome medical facts at didactics (medical lectures on Wednesday afternoons). This may not sound like fun, but it was nice to get a break for a few hours (albeit spotted with answering pages between speakers) from hospital work.

9. Ros, Lisa, Maria, Mary Ann, Dian and all the other Family Health Center nurses and staff — hugs, love, laughs.

10. Free lunch three days a week while on Floors.

11. Fancy dinners throughout recruitment season. I miss those steaks.

12. Evening office hours. Just like being on call, working odd hours created a cozy camaraderie. We would relax and laugh more. We were already working into the evening; who needed to rush?

13. Having an attending available if I wasn't sure about a clinical decision. At any moment, there was an attending a phone call away if I really needed support.

14. Knowing that in three years, regardless of how bad it was, everything would change.

APPENDIX B: HOW JUDE AND I STAYED TOGETHER

1. We maintained regular physical intimacy. Because of fatigue and my grueling schedule, I didn't have much of a libido. When I had the slightest desire for sex, we acted on it, even if it was only once a month. But even if we didn't have sex, we showed affection emotionally and physically. The power of touch is so healing and helped us stay close.

2. We made an effort to be there for each other — in sad times as well as happy times...and on boring days in between.

3. I gave Jude a detailed list of my weekly schedule. This helped in making future plans. My calendar was color-coded. Things that couldn't be moved were in pink. These included office hours, call nights and date night.

4. We wrote our thoughts in our own journals. This helped to clear our minds of worries and concerns and eased the emotional burden on each other. When I had time, I would go out alone to a coffee shop and write in my journal.

5. I avoided taking moonlighting shifts if possible. Moonlighting is *extra* work outside the residency. Although it may sound crazy, it was tempting to take

these shifts because they pay $45 to $75 an hour, compared with regular residency shifts, which pay only about $8 to $13 an hour, depending on the program. Even so, I took only two moonlighting shifts. The hours I could have made more money were more valuable as sleep time or to spend time with Jude.

6. We made an effort to take short weekend trips together when we could. We did this on Golden Weekends, which came about once a month. The change of scenery allowed some distance between us and residency and helped us to refocus.

7. We kept activities simple. Sometimes taking a walk together was the most helpful, healing thing we could do. Still is.

8. I invited Jude to visit me when I was on call for a few extra minutes of time together.

9. We scheduled time at least once or twice a week to talk about my work. My instinct was *not* to talk about it; I thought it was more important to hear about Jude's day, and to distract myself. But being in complete denial of 80 percent of my life was destructive, and talking about it with her kept us close.

10. We cherished time spent together. Jude and I both realized that the bottom could fall out at any second, that our friends' relationships were undergoing constant change, and that we needed to treasure time together to keep ourselves together.

11. We followed the rules. Before I met Jude and we became committed, I would have said that relationship "rules" were silly. Nonetheless, after trial and error, we gradually created a few guidelines that helped keep things simple

and cut down on petty arguments and worry. Here they are:

a. The "10" Rule: Prevents resentment and honors each person's values. If I want to go to a concert on Friday night, and I will resent anything or anyone that gets in my way, I just say, "I'm a 10 on the concert Friday." And then Jude knows I am serious, and doesn't offer other plans. We go to the concert, because she knows it is really important to me. Voila, no resentment. *Caveat — do not overuse the 10. Respect the 10.

b. The No Directives Rule: Prevents resentment. Jude and I agreed on this in the first month we were dating. Essentially, it says, "Don't tell me what to do." This sentiment is fairly universal...people don't like to be dominated by command statements. "Give me that." "Stop that." "Get out of the car." "Get more sleep." These types of comments feel awkward in any case. They are appropriate for parents to give their young children, from superior to inferior officer in military operations and in immediately dangerous situations (e.g. "Stop the car! Watch out for that hippo!"). However, in personal relationships, they seem to breed annoyance if not outright hostility.

c. The Six-Month Rule: Prevents bad or rash decision-making and life ruts. Jude once visited a pig farm. She then wanted to be a pig farmer. Later, I thought it would be a good idea to drop out of residency and start a cemetery business. Maybe these would've been good life changes, but probably not. The Six-Month Rule states that if you want to make a major life change (get a new job, move to a new city, have kids, get a facial tattoo, break up), then that person must want that major life change for six consecutive months. At the end, if you still want to do it, the two of you make the change together.

d. The Beep Rule: Prevents petty arguments regarding decision-making. We sometimes had arguments for no reason whatsoever. So now, if one of us doesn't care at all, they can 'beep.' For example:

"What do you want to do for dinner?"

"I don't know, what do you want to do?"

"I don't care...what do you think?"

"Well, we could always make spaghetti."

"Yeah, but we had that last night."

"Well, I really don't care. You pick."

"No, I picked last night."

And on, and on.

This rule states that if you truly do not care, you may say "Beep" and be completely let off the hook for the decision. It also means that the other party is required to make the decision, and that you may not complain about the decision, nor offer other ideas.

12. We are finding ourselves. Now that residency is over, Jude and I are untangling our codependent relationship to find ourselves again. We had to hold each other up for years and bury many emotionally heavy problems. We are each seeing therapists who are helping us reshape our lives and unpack all the baggage. We can do this.

GLOSSARY

Attending: A resident's boss. A "real" doctor.

BCMS: A.k.a. Big City Medical Student. Medical trainees who are smart and willing to do anything for brownie points from attendings.

Boards: A series of many tests throughout medical school, residency and every seven years thereafter. When passed, the physician is then deemed "Board Certified."

Call: Scheduled after-hours medical work. This varies based upon years of training. During Shadyside's first and second years of residency, these hours are spent "in-house," meaning physically in the hospital.

ERAS (Electronic Residency Application Service): An organization that matches medical students (for a fee) with residency programs in a process called "The Match."

Intern: A first-year resident, usually right out of medical school.

MCAT (Medical College Admission Test): Exam taken by pre-med students to gain acceptance to medical school.

Medical School (aka med school): Four-year medical training after college and before residency. The first two years are usually classroom/lecture-based; the last two are like apprenticeships, working directly with other physicians (called rotations).

Moonlighting: Extra work in a hospital, above and beyond residency. Pays well. Shifts usually last five to 12 hours.

Pimping (i.e., Pimp Session): When a senior physician grills a junior physician or med student with medical questions, often in the presence of the junior physician's peers. The purpose for this varies — it can be a tool to teach the junior physician, to teach the group of junior physicians, to establish hierarchy or to shame the junior physician.

Residency: A period of training (three-plus years) between medical school and The Real World.

Resident: A doctor who is in training, after graduating from medical school. There are two types of residents: interns (first-year residents) and seniors (second-year and beyond).

Rotations: A succession of month-long periods during medical school and residency, when doctors study a single specialty (i.e., general surgery, gynecology or Floors) in a hospital setting.

Rounding: A period, usually one to three hours in the morning, when physicians take care of patients in the hospital. Sometimes it's done individually (attending, resident, intern, medical student each independently round, then discuss), sometimes as a team.

Secondaries: The second part of the long application process to get into med school (usually an essay and another fee).

Sign-out/sign-in: Quickly passing on patient information from one shift-worker to the next.

BIBLIOGRAPHY

AAFP. (2015). *Family Medicine Facts*. Retrieved from American Academy of Family Physicians: http://www.aafp.org/about/the-aafp/family-medicine-facts.html

Blosser, F. (2005, January 13). *Medical Interns' Risk for Car Crashes Linked With Extended Shifts in NIOSH-Funded Study*. Retrieved from Centers for Disease Control and Prevention: http://www.cdc.gov/niosh/updates/upd-01-13-05.html

College, P. a. (2010). Harvard Health Publications. Harvard Health Publications.

Fostick, L. B. (June 2014, Vol 57(3)). Effect of 24 Hours of Sleep Deprivation on Auditory and Linguistic Perception: A Comparison among Young Controls, Sleep-Deprived Participants, Dyslexic Readers, and Aging Adults. *Journal of Speech, Language & Hearing Research*, 1078-1088.

Keller, P. S. (Vol 23(4), 2014). Sleep Deprivation and Dating Aggression Perpetration in Female College Students: The Moderating Roles of Trait Aggression, Victimization by Partner, and Alcohol Use. *Journal of Aggression, Maltreatment & Trauma*, 3.

Peckham, C. (2015, January 26). *Medscape Physician Lifestyle Report*. Retrieved from Medscape: http://www.medscape.com/features/slideshow/lifestyle/2015/public/overview

Pilcher, J. J. (Vol 19(4), May 1996). Effects of Sleep Deprivation on Performance: A meta-analysis. *Sleep: Journal of Sleep Research & Sleep Medicine*, 318-326.

Sinha, P. (2014, September 4). Retrieved from NY Times: http://www.nytimes.com/2014/09/05/opinion/why-do-doctors-commit-suicide.html?_r=0

Skertich, T. (2010). *Adventures in Medicine: The Resident's Guide to Life and Practice*.

Vandale, K. (Vol 166(2)). Sleep Deprivation in EMS. *Fire Fighting*, 18-25.